PEOPLE a]

C000061177

Homoeopathy for first-time users and their pets

by
Francis Hunter
MRCVS, VetMFHom
and
Steven Kayne
**PhD, MRPharmS, DAgVetPharm,
MPS(NZ), LFHom (Pharm)**

Cartoons by Roğ

Published by
The British Homoeopathic Association
27A Devonshire Street, London, W1N 1RJ

© 1997 British Homoeopathic Association

First published in 1997 by
British Homoeopathic Association,
27A Devonshire Street,
London, W1N 1RJ

A charity registered in England No. 235900

British Library Cataloguing in Publication Data.
A catalogue record for this book is available from the British Library.

ISBN No. 0 946717 71 0

DEDICATION

TO PEOPLE (AND THEIR PETS), WHOEVER AND
WHEREVER THEY ARE, IN THE HOPE THAT, BY
READING THIS SIMPLE BOOK, THEY WILL BE
INTRODUCED TO HOMOEOPATHY, A GENTLE AND
VERY EFFECTIVE FORM OF TREATMENT FOR
MANY INJURIES AND ILLNESSES.

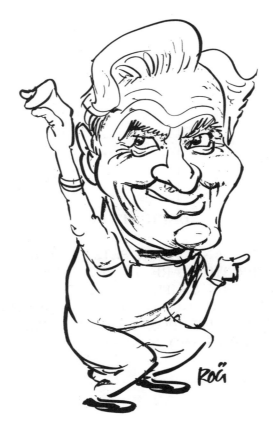

Francis Hunter is Chairman of the British Homoeopathic Association and a founder member of the British Association of Homoeopathic Veterinary Surgeons, serving as its President from 1993-1996. Since his retirement from a busy Sussex practice, he runs a part-time referral service treating animals with homoeopathy or acupuncture.

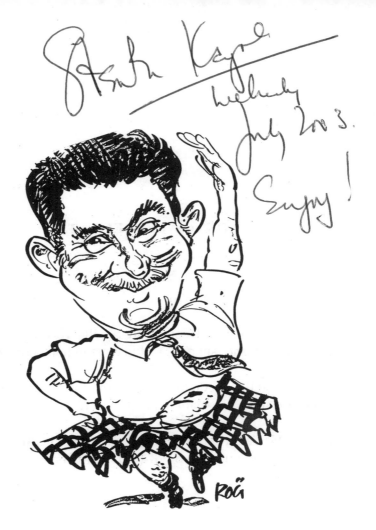

Dr Steven Kayne is a community pharmacist in Glasgow. He lectures and writes widely on homoeopathy both in the UK and abroad. He is Pharmacy Tutor to the Faculty of Homoeopathy, in London and Glasgow, and visiting lecturer in complementary medicine at the University of Strathclyde, Glasgow.

ACKNOWLEDGEMENTS

We wish to thank the following:

Our wives, Yvonne Hunter and Sorelle Kayne, for their constant help and support, and interest in homoeopathy.

Enid Segall, Secretary General of the British Homoeopathic Association, and her staff.

Linda McCann, who edited our whole effort into chronological order and proof-read the final copy, ready for publication.

CONTENTS

FOREWORD

by
Katie Boyle

It's great that Francis Hunter and Steven Kayne have joined forces but, if ever a book needed no foreword, this is it!

It already has an informative preface in the light-hearted exchange between the two authors; then comes an introduction which includes details of homoeopathic source materials. I've always wondered about some of these!

But "People are Pets" is far more than an introduction to homoeopathy.

Ever since my cradle days, I was treated most effectively with many of these remedies but, as I grew up, I became aware that, whilst our homoeopathic practitioner in Rapallo (where we had a villa and spent our summers), the Dottoressa Bacigalupo, was always in demand, her husband, a charming and allopathic pharmacist, was equally popular and their chemist-shop was well-stocked with both homoeopathic and conventional choices.

"Whatever works best in the different circumstances, we use", I often heard both husband and wife say and it is the same sentence I've heard frequently from Francis Hunter. I can't remember a time when I haven't been in close touch with Francis, and his brilliant choice of remedies has dotted our relationship.

Two cases, in particular, are
1) his choice of 2 daily tablets of *Bufo rana* (poison of a toad - preferably Mexican, he tells me!). These I give to my Italian greyhound, who was diagnosed as epileptic a few years ago, (no Phenobarbitone for her) and *Bufo rana* has kept her free of fits ever since.
2) 8 daily drops of *Haronga* (the bark of a Madagascan shrub) which, combined with a fat-free diet, curb my toy poodle's pancreatitis very successfully. These are just two of his successes but I could list a great many more.

The Francis Hunter/Steven Kayne team is great and it is their knowledgeable, but easy-read, approach linked very amusingly by Roǧ's cartoons that make "People are Pets" a book to keep close at hand.

I'll dip into it frequently and hope a great many people will do the same. We'll all have fun whilst learning a lot.

PREFACE

The British Homoeopathic Association took a stand at a recent SAGA Lifestyle Festival, which Francis helped to man, in order, it was thought, to answer questions about homoeopathy for people's pets but it transpired that not many of the visitors to the show owned pets any more. However, when asked the question, "do you have a pet at home?", the frequent reply was, "no, not now, this is my only pet", as they, rather charmingly, put their arm around their companion. Hence, people, as well as animals, can be pets and so the title of this book evolved!

At the present time, there is an ever-increasing interest and demand for all forms of complementary or, if you prefer the term, alternative medicine. The British Homoeopathic Association, whose principal aim is to promote homoeopathy, felt that there was a need for a simple, easy to follow, short, illustrated book that could be of use to the whole family, embracing any household pets, animal or human. The main object, therefore, is to present homoeopathy in a straightforward, light-hearted manner in order to try and interest new readers in this gentle, yet very effective, form of treatment.

Treatments for humans and pets are very similar, according to the following conversation between our authors:

Steven: Are there any major differences in the way in which you practise homoeopathy for animals, Francis, from the way in which it is used to treat humans?

Francis:	No, I think the procedures are very similar.
Steven:	Well, you say that, but how can it be? You are using remedies on the basis of the way in which they are used in humans. But fish and birds and cows and sheep are completely different to humans.
Francis:	All creatures are made up of cells or cellular tissue and homoeopathy seems to work at a cell level.
Steven:	So, are you convinced that it works on animals?
Francis:	The undeniable proof, here, is that the animals have no idea what medicine they are receiving and if there is an improvement, or even a slight reaction, then it must be due to the remedy and not a placebo-effect, as is often argued for humans.
Steven:	So, we are going to use the anecdotes as a means of explaining how remedies can be used. Is that the idea?
Francis:	I think we both feel that the book has a serious purpose but that, by presenting it in a light-hearted way with the cartoons and anecdotes, we hope that it will appeal to a wide readership who know little, or nothing, about homoeopathy.

WHAT IS HOMOEOPATHY?

Homoeopathy is the administration of minute quantities of medicines that, in much greater concentration, actually cause symptoms similar to those being treated. This concept is often summarised in the phrase 'let like be treated by like'.

Perhaps the most important feature of homoeopathy is its holistic approach to healing. This means that practitioners base their choice of remedy on **all** aspects of a patient's health, rather than just on the symptoms alone.

Generations of people (and pets!) have found it both safe and effective in treating many different problems.

Homoeopathy and related non-orthodox treatments, such as medical herbalism, aromatherapy, and the manipulative techniques (e.g. chiropractic and osteopathy), are often called 'alternative medicine'. This term implies that one has to choose one of two courses of action. For example, making decisions between orthodox medicine and homoeopathy, or between homoeopathy and nothing.

In fact, it is the **complementary** approach that is to be favoured. Here, it is possible to complement, or complete, what is already available, using the most appropriate combination of treatments in any given set of circumstances. It may well be that an orthodox medicine and a homoeopathic medicine could be used together to treat different aspects of the same disease. Antibiotics are often prescribed with *Belladonna* by medically qualified homoeopathic physicians. Equally, there may be

1

circumstances under which either type of medicine is inappropriate and the use of the other method of treatment can prove very valuable.

Good examples, for using homoeopathy, are in pregnancy (for morning sickness), or where there are fears of interactions in taking preparations, like travel sickness tablets or anti-diarrhoeals, by patients already being treated with prescription medication. Treatment of 'exam nerves' or 'show-ring fright' in animals are other examples.

HOMOEOPATHY - THE EARLY YEARS

Britain played an important part in the development of homoeopathy, the complementary medical discipline, pioneered by Christian Samuel Hahnemann. He was born in Saxony, eastern Germany, in 1755. While translating a textbook by the great Scottish physician, William Cullen, Dr Hahnemann found himself in disagreement regarding the action of quinine, a recently introduced remedy for a condition, then called marsh fever, but now known as malaria. He tested the drug on himself by taking relatively large amounts and recording every physical and mental symptom that resulted. In this way, he was able to produce a comprehensive 'drug-picture'. Remarkably, this was very similar to the symptom-picture reported by patients suffering from malaria.

Hahnemann also observed that the symptoms of *Belladonna* poisoning were similar to those of scarlet fever, for which the remedy was being prescribed at that time. He claimed a law of drug action suggesting that

2

remedies producing certain symptoms in healthy persons could cure sick persons presenting with similar symptoms.

Britain's first Homoeopath was Dr F.J. Harvey Quin, who qualified from Edinburgh Medical School in 1820.

THE THREE PRINCIPLES OF HOMOEOPATHY

1) Like to treat like:

This first principle is embodied in the phrase 'Similia similibus curentur' or 'let like be treated by like'. Examples might be the use of *Coffea* (coffee) (see page 99), to treat insomnia, or *Apis mel.* (from the bee) (see page 24), to treat stings and similar histamine-type reactions.

At first sight, this is rather different to the orthodox approach, when the use of Syrup of Figs to treat diarrhoea might cause a few eyebrows to be raised! However, there are several examples of this practice in orthodox medicine.

Above a certain dose level, the drug digoxin causes many of the heart conditions for which it is also a treatment; aspirin, in large doses, causes headaches.

2) The minimal dose:

When Hahnemann did his original work, he administered substantial doses of medicine to his patients, not always with good results. Subsequently, he experimented by diluting his remedies and found that, as the concentration fell, remarkably the therapeutic effect rose.

It is in this area where many people have extreme difficulty in accepting that homoeopathic remedies can possibly work. Much is made of the huge dilutions that are involved in some homoeopathic treatments when, theoretically, there are no molecules of remedy left in solution that can be detected with the methods we have available today.

However, homoeopathy is not only about these huge dilutions. Potencies such as 6c, a 1 in 100 serial dilution carried out 6 times with fierce bursts of agitation (see 'Preparing the remedy', page 8), are used frequently, particularly over the counter in pharmacies and, at this level, there are still molecules left in solution. Quantities of drug present are of the same order of normally prescribed amounts of many orthodox medicines; for example, thyroxine.

3) The single remedy:

Hahnemann's final idea was that of using a single remedy to treat patients' ills although, in later life, he did administer more than one remedy concurrently. Indeed, the appearance of mixtures of remedies has proved popular, in modern times, although classical homoeopaths frown on the practice. Many of us would welcome the demise of medicines with numerous ingredients!

To these three important principles, we can add the idea of the holistic approach - **treating the whole person**. The holistic approach to treatment is, perhaps, the most important concept, within the practice of homoeopathy, and is shared with all other complementary disciplines.

To a homoeopath, there is no one remedy for an illness. One remedy may be used to treat a wide range of different conditions in different patients, and two patients with similar symptoms may not receive the same remedy. The aim is to restore a patient (or pet) to his or her own unique state of 'wellness', taking into account any environmental influences, and not just to an 'average' well state.

A first consultation, for a long-standing condition, might take 30-40 minutes, during which time the patient will be asked all sorts of seemingly unrelated questions about their personality and environmental preferences. In this way, the practitioner can build up a total picture of the patient before considering any symptoms that prompted the visit. Rather than treating the case as 'a sore throat attached to a body', a prescription will be issued on the basis of 'a body with a sore throat'.

Without some knowledge, the beginner would find it difficult to treat complicated long-standing illnesses, and this limits the conditions that can be realistically treated by self-medication.

However, luckily, there is a range of around 20 'specifics' or **polychrests**; remedies with wide applications that can be used routinely to help many common ailments and first aid situations. In the main, it is these remedies that are described in this book.

THE SOURCE MATERIAL

More than 50% of all remedies are prepared from plant extracts and, because of this, homoeopathy is often confused with herbalism by many people.

The original work carried out by Hahnemann, used naturally occurring chemicals together with their trace impurities as well as vegetable material. Thus, the remedy *Calc. carb.* (chalk) is obtained from the interspaces of oysters and is not prepared in the laboratory. *Sulphur* comes from geothermal areas. Animal and insect material must be obtained from healthy specimens. *Lactrodectus* is a spider, whose venom is sometimes used in the treatment of the heart condition, angina.

Finally, there is a mixed bag of source material including mixed pollens, house dust and house dust mites, flowers, cat and dog hair, feathers and various foods. Remedies prepared from these sources are said to be 'isopathic' and involve something akin to vaccination therapy, treating 'same with same' as opposed to classical homoeopathy, when 'like is treated with like'.

PREPARING THE REMEDY

Mother Tinctures are liquid preparations resulting from the extraction of suitable source material, with alcohol/water mixtures, and form the starting point for the production of most homoeopathic medicines.

With insoluble chemicals, such as *Sulphur* (and many of the isopathic preparations mentioned above), the solid material must be ground down ('triturated') with lactose powder, using a pestle and mortar, in a precise and documented manner. The process must be carried out in a warm, dry atmosphere with perfectly clean equipment.

The resulting triturate may be compressed directly into **trituration tablets**, or administered as a powder if the remedy is required at potencies where it is still insoluble. More usually, however, trituration continues until the

6

particle size has been reduced sufficiently to facilitate the preparation of a solution.

With some remedies, for example *Arnica* or *Calendula*, the mother tincture may be applied directly to the skin, or it may be diluted and used as a gargle; *Crataegus* mother tincture, for heart problems, is often administered as five drops in water.

Most other mother tinctures, however, are diluted in a very special manner. Because this dilution increases the homoeopathic strength, the process is known as **potentisation or dynamisation**.

The **Hahnemannian method of potentisation** provides two scales of dilution, 'centesimal' and 'decimal'. In the former, one drop of mother tincture is added to 99 drops of diluent in a new, clean screw-cap glass vial. The diluent is an alcohol and water mixture, the strength of which varies from 20% to 60%. For accuracy, the 99 drops are usually measured with a special calibrated glass pipette.

The solution, resulting from a mixture of the two liquids, is subjected to a vigorous shaking, with impact, known as **succussion**. In Hahnemann's day, the procedure was effected by striking the vial on a large leather-bound book, typically the family Bible. Nowadays, in a more secular environment, the same effect is usually obtained with a special mechanical shaker! There are many pharmacists who still succuss by hand, striking the vial on the heel of their palms. The extent, to which the vials are shaken, depends on the individual concerned; somewhere between 20 and 40 times is often quoted as being appropriate.

After the initial process, successive serial dilutions follow, using fresh glass vials at each stage, until the solution reaches 12c, 30c, 200c, and so on; the number refers to the number of successive 1 in 100 dilutions and 'c' indicates the centesimal method. The letter 'c' is sometimes left out when describing the potency.

Very high dilutions are usually expressed with roman numerals. Thus, 1,000c is denoted simply by the letter 'M', the small letter 'c' being implied. A 10,000 potency (i.e. a 1 in 100 dilution carried out serially 10,000 times) is denoted by 10M. There are some ultra high potencies- CM (100,000), MM (1000,000) and even higher, but these are seldom used.

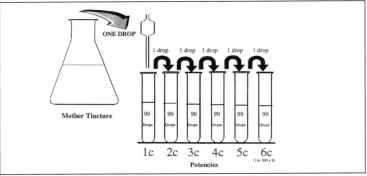

Fig 1. *Diagram to illustrate the serial dilution process*

The decimal dilution method is similar, except that the process involves adding one drop to nine drops of diluent. The potencies are designated by a number with the letter 'x' following it. Thus, 6x represents a 1 in 10 dilution carried out serially 6 times, each with a burst of succussion.

8

Dilution on a grand scale or, as some unkind critics have suggested, placing 5mls of drug solution at the source of a river and collecting it downstream, will not work because of the lack of succussion. It is for this reason that fluoridisation of the water supply is not homoeopathically active, although the chemical is present in homoeopathic amounts.

We do not know why the potentisation process is so important. Some homoeopaths suggest that it is merely a way of ensuring the dilutions are thoroughly mixed, while others suggest that some energy is imparted, to the solution, in the shaking process. Like much of homoeopathy, the explanation still eludes us.

When a solution has been obtained, at the required potency, it can be used to prepare the appropriate dose form. This may be tablets, pills, powders, liquids, ointments, creams and lotions.

HOW DO HOMOEOPATHIC REMEDIES WORK?

There have been numerous suggestions as to how homoeopathic remedies might work but, as yet, we have no definitive explanation. However, there are precedents for medicines to be used without understanding their mode of action, in orthodox medicine. For example, British sailors were given limes to suck by the great Scottish naval surgeon, Lind, in the 18th century, to prevent scurvy. This was based on empirical observations - it was nearly 200 years before the link between scurvy and vitamin C deficiency was fully unravelled.

There is no doubt that homoeopathy suffers from an inability to provide scientific evidence as to how it works. The discipline has evolved as a patient-orientated therapy, based on clinical observation rather than on scientific principles. Sceptics use this fact as a basis for their comments. "Homoeopathy cannot possibly work," they say. But those of us who use homoeopathy daily in our practices know that it does!

Homoeopaths consider disease to be an expression of a person's vital force, a vibrating dynamic element, called 'physis' by Hippocrates from which came the term 'physician'. According to the theories of vitalism, the body comprises cells, tissues, and organs that are fully interdependent and whose relationship to one another is controlled by a steering entity - the vital force. If this force becomes disturbed by factors, such as stress, poor diet or environmental conditions, illness will result. The homoeopath seeks to normalise the vital force, with the help of remedies, thus encouraging the body to heal itself.

RESEARCH

Despite the existence of many research papers and media exposure, homoeopathy continues to suffer from an inability to explain its action scientifically. A lack of human and financial resources is hampering progress, at present, but interesting work in human and veterinary areas is proceeding, not only to prove efficacy but to improve our methods of administration. Methods of proving effectiveness, based on patients' own perceptions (rather than on scientific evidence), are now being developed in Glasgow.

HOMOEOPATHY IN THE COMMUNITY

It is probably true to say that most health professionals, involved in the provision of homoeopathic services, have adopted a reactive approach, seeking to satisfy a demand from the public that has intensified over recent years. However, with professional training, this is changing and there has been a significant increase in the number of NHS, private, and veterinary homoeopathic prescriptions presented by patients, as a result of a more proactive approach.

Over the last ten years, the number of people using homoeopathy has more than doubled to 28% of the population, with a similar percentage saying that they would now consider the discipline.

The reasons for people turning to homoeopathy are interesting to speculate. Many patients perceive homoeopathy as attracting much less risk than orthodox medicines, with an absence of side effects; others may be dissatisfied with the treatment received from orthodox GPs, and see homoeopathic physicians as having more time to discuss their problems in a caring manner; others may be impressed by the Royal connection, or have found orthodox medicines ineffective. Immigrant communities may have a traditional mistrust of Western medicine.

Critics of homoeopathy base most of their arguments on the lack of scientific evidence. This does not seem to trouble our Euro cousins on the other side of the Channel. If a remedy can be shown to be safe and efficacious, they will use it, despite a lack of understanding of its mechanisms.

There are lots of examples of orthodox, or 'allopathic', medicines whose action we do not fully understand - some, like paracetamol, are not as safe as homoeopathic remedies. Further, such proof of efficacy does not seem to apply to the various preparations, including cough mixtures, that have been prescribed, over the counter, for years despite doubtful efficacy.

The UK homoeopathic market (worth about £16m, annually) pales into insignificance if one takes a look at the market in other EC countries. In France, for example, with a population similar to ours, homoeopathy has a market value of about 15 times the UK. In the Netherlands, the average spending on homoeopathy, per head of population, in 1995 was around £5.50, compared with around £0.25 here. The figures are not entirely compatible, for a series of reasons, but even if appropriate adjustments could be made, there would still be a large disparity.

LEVELS OF TREATMENT AND DOSE REGIMES

1) Common potencies

The most common strength, or **potency**, of homoeopathic medicine, available 'over the counter' in pharmacies and health stores in the UK, is probably the 6c. As can be seen from *fig. 1* (see page 8), this represents a dilution of 1 in 100, repeated 6 times. The potency 30c is also available widely.

Homoeopaths are divided as to which potency is the more appropriate in different sets of circumstances. We will apply our comments to both the 6c and 30c potencies in this book.

Do consult your vet, doctor, pharmacist or health store assistant for advice on the use of other potencies.

2) Dose

It has been shown that sufficient active medicine is present in one tablet to treat both adults and children even though, often, you will see the dose as being two tablets for an adult and one for children. Animals can be given tablets on the same basis.

Each dose should be given at least half an hour before food or after a meal.

3) Frequency

In contrast with orthodox medicine, in homoeopathy, it is the *frequency* of dose that is more important than the size of the dose. The choice of dose frequency depends on whether the treatment is considered to be first aid, acute, or chronic.

13

In the context of the book, we may define the terms as follows:

a) First aid: This is the first, or initial, treatment given when the condition is first identified, rather than the traditional understanding of the term as being treatment for an accidental injury. It, thus, includes treatment for the first signs of a cold or fever. Homoeopathic medicines are administered, frequently, under these circumstances - perhaps as often as every 5-15 minutes for 6 doses at either 6c or 30c potency levels.

The first aid (or 'first treatment') remedies are very effective, with clear indications for use, and the response can be seen within minutes. The remedy *Aconite* (see page 21) might be used, at this level, when the first symptoms of a cold appear. It can also be given for fright. *Arnica* (see page 30) may be given, this frequently, after a fall, or collision, resulting in bruising. When troublesome symptoms persist, dosing can be continued on the acute scale.

b) Acute: Acute treatment is administered for a condition that is beyond its initial stages and is now causing relatively severe symptoms, that are likely to be of limited duration. Examples might include diarrhoea or a cough.

With acute prescribing, it is necessary to seek a little more information than with the first aid approach (where a single symptom is usually enough) in order to choose the most appropriate remedy.

Each remedy has a number of 'keynotes', indicating its main use, on which administration can be based. In order to differentiate between remedies with similar uses, and to individualise treatment, it may be necessary to seek answers to questions concerning **modalities** (see page 17).

The treatment of acute conditions involves taking the 6c potency, 3 or 4 times a day, or the 30c potency, 2 or 3 times daily. The acute phase of an illness may last up to 10 days but, often, a major improvement will occur within 24-48 hours. If this is the case, dosing can be discontinued earlier.

A sudden cold might be treated in this way if intervention at the first aid level, during the initial stages, was not possible or ineffective.

In the 'over the counter' situation, it is often recommended that a complete course of treatment, extending over several days, is taken but, where a patient (human or animal) is being treated directly by a homoeopathic practitioner, this pattern may be varied, according to individual responses.

c) Chronic: Here, we are talking about conditions such as a troublesome cough, that drags on for weeks, or a soft tissue injury, such as a strain or sprain. It must be emphasised that we are not talking about long-standing problems, like heart disease or breathing difficulties, that should not be self-treated, without professional advice.

Chronic remedies require more than the simple first aid or acute approach mentioned above: modalities are important (see page 17).

In chronic self-treatment, the patient is normally advised to take the 6c remedy, twice daily for 4-6 weeks, before reviewing the situation, except where **aggravation** is experienced (see page 18).

4) The constitutional remedy

One very specialised application of homoeopathy involves the administration of constitutional remedies. We mention them, here, in case you should hear them discussed and wonder what they are.

In any group of people, clinical experience tells us that some patients will respond especially well to a particular remedy. Amongst this sub-group, certain physical and mental characteristics appear to be common (eg. hair colour, skin tone, or a tendency to cry easily) and, often, they may reflect the characteristics of the remedy too. We talk about these groups as being 'constitutional types'.

Pulsatilla (wind-flower) is an example of a constitutional remedy. *Pulsatilla* people are said to have a changeable disposition and this reflects the nature of the plant, from which the remedy is made, so named because it sways in the wind from side to side.

It is possible to identify constitutional types amongst animals. The Irish setter is said to respond well to the remedy made from the element, red *Phosphorus* and, indeed, it might be expected that this was so, as it has been found that red-headed people have an affinity for this remedy.

Most of the 15 common constitutional remedies are also polychrests. They are used to improve general well-being and to assist in some other forms of homoeopathic treatment. For best effect, one needs to know a lot about the patient - and a lot about the remedy too. We do not recommend their use without further study.

MODALITIES

'Better for' and 'worse for' symptoms are very important to homoeopaths. They are known as modalities.

The homoeopathic remedies, *Rhus tox.*(see page 83) and *Bryonia*, (see page 40) can both be used to treat rheumatic-type conditions in human or veterinary patients. However, patients who find relief from wrapping an ice pack around their joints, and for whom any sort of movement is extremely painful, seem to respond better to *Bryonia*. Patients, who find that the application of warmth to the affected part is beneficial, and for whom initial movement is painful but continuing movement acceptable, find *Rhus tox.* helpful.

This differentiation of symptoms would not normally be considered in orthodox medicine; it is probable that all rheumatic patients would be given similar analgesics or non-steroidal anti-inflammatory drugs.

Examples of common modalities are:
- Site: Pain better or worse, on the right or left side of the body.
- Time: Pain better or worse, at night or in the morning, certain seasons or times of the month.

17

- Environmental: Pain better or worse in cold/hot weather.
- Temperature: Pain better or worse for the application of heat/cold.

Such information allows us to make the most appropriate choice from several potential remedies. Modalities have been included in most of the abbreviated drug pictures given in this book. Because people are not used to identifying such things as a 'left sided sore throat', they generally do not volunteer the information without prompting. Asking the right questions is often the key to successful **repertorisation** - the process of matching symptoms to an appropriate remedy.

In some books, the symbols < and > are used to signify aggravation ('worse for') and amelioration ('better for') respectively.

AGGRAVATION

Aggravation is said to occur when the condition being treated becomes marginally worse, and is considered to be a positive indication. It happens in about 10% of cases, usually appearing within 2-5 days of commencing the first treatment.

Dosing should be discontinued until the symptoms fall back to their original intensity (2-3 days). The remedy should then be restarted, but at a lower frequency, i.e. once a day instead of twice a day.

TAKING THE REMEDY

Homoeopathic remedies are rather different from orthodox medicines in the way in which they are taken. The active ingredients are carried on the surface of the solid dose forms (tablets, granules, etc) and should not be handled any more than absolutely necessary.

The best way of taking medicine is to tip the required amount into the cap of the container and then transfer it into the mouth. Humans should allow the remedy to dissolve in the mouth; it is acknowledged that this may be difficult to achieve with pets.

Peppermint is thought to inactivate homoeopathic remedies and highly flavoured toothpaste should be replaced by a bland variety, if possible. It is often reported that patients should avoid tea and coffee, but restricting oneself to 4-5 cups a day, and observing the 'half-hour' rule, should be sufficient precautions.

STORAGE

The remedies should not be mixed with other remedies. They should be kept in their original container with a tightly fitting cap.

Ideally, they should be packed in glass but, for short courses of treatment, plastic is quite acceptable for solid dose forms (granules, pills, tablets etc). The remedies should be stored away from direct light and great heat and they should not be exposed to aromatic odours.

To satisfy the medicines' regulations, an expiry date of two years may be put on the label. In fact, there is circumstantial evidence that remedies retain their therapeutic activity for many years.

GUIDELINES FOR DOSING DOGS AND CATS

1) Dogs: Tablets are slightly sweet and, for this reason, the dog will often chew them or lick them off a clean spoon.

Alternatively, they can be dropped into the animal's mouth or crushed to a powder in a fold of clean paper. If the animal will only take the dose with food, the medicine can be put in a small morsel of bread or some favourite treat.

2) Cats: Medicines can be given, as for dogs. If necessary, the tablets can be powdered and mixed with a very small amount of butter. This mixture can then be placed directly in the cat's mouth, or on its front paws, when it will be licked off quickly. Individual powders and granules are also used; in the latter case, a dose is represented by a 'small pinch'.

It can be easier to administer your pet's remedy in liquid form. Two or three drops of liquid remedy can be added to your pet's drinking water. The animal, thus, doses itself several times during the day. This is important, in first aid situations, because animals' metabolic rates are higher than humans and they often require more frequent dosing.

ACONITE (Aconitum napellus)

Aconite, known as monk's-hood or wolf's-bane, is a member of the Ranunculaceae or buttercup family. The whole plant is extremely poisonous but when it has been made into a homoeopathic medicine, by dilution and succussion (see page 7-10), all the poisonous or 'bad bits' have been removed, leaving only the 'good' or 'healing' properties.

It is appropriate that this is the first remedy to talk about in this book. *Aconite* is the remedy to think of first in any situation where there is shock, such as accidents, fear, bleeding, and also where the development of a fever appears imminent. It is a very quick acting remedy (its effects are noticeable in minutes) but it is also short-acting and, therefore, may need repeating several times, even within an hour.

Keynotes: Shock, fast action.

Uses: *Aconite* may be used in cases of fear, shock, injury, or wounds with bleeding, as already indicated above. *Aconite* can steady the nerves after an accident or unexpected event, such as a road traffic accident or a fall, and may be invaluable also in helping to control pain of any kind. It is a very useful remedy at the beginning of a fever, such as influenza, or tonsillitis, sudden high temperature, or, in the case of animals, the early stages of 'kennel cough' etc.

Modalities: Better in the open air, worse in a warm room, and in the evening. Worse lying on the affected side.

Suggested Potency: 30c.

Dosage: Every 5-15 minutes up to 6 doses, if necessary, until the condition begins to settle down. There is no harm in continuing with doses of *Aconite* for longer, if the situation seems to demand it, but it often seems appropriate, after a few doses of *Aconite*, to change to a different selected remedy according to the symptom picture.

Additional Remedies: *Arnica* (see page 30) is also a shock remedy and often follows *Aconite* well. *Sulphur* (see page 90), in chronic cases, may help to complete a cure started with *Aconite*. *Coffea* (see page 99) is also useful, if there is extreme excitability.

Anecdote: I am often reminded of a 'picture' portrayed in a lecture given by the well-known homoeopathic physician, Dr Jack, some years ago. He told us of moving down a bus distributing *Aconite* tablets to all the passengers after a road traffic accident, whilst awaiting the arrival of an ambulance, and how it helped to calm people. (FH)

ACONITE

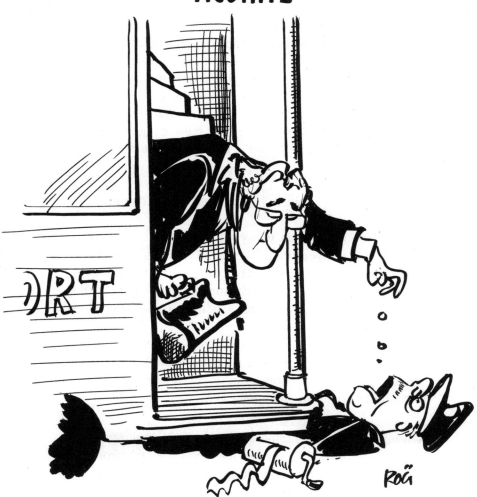

APIS MEL. (Apis mellifica)

Apis mel. is prepared from the honey bee. The venom from the bee has been used in folklore, since early times, for its medicinal properties, but in fact it seems that the whole insect, rather than just the poison from the sting, contains constituents that are useful in the homoeopathic medicine and, so, the 'mother tincture' contains the whole dead insect.

This remedy neatly sums up the basis of homoeopathic medicine; that is, that 'what a substance can cause it can also cure'.

Keynotes: Stings, bites. Severe swelling. Oedema.

Uses: This remedy, in many ways, acts like the modern diuretic of conventional medicine and is capable of removing excess fluids from the tissues. Its indications for use, therefore, are all kinds of stings and bites which cause sudden and painful swellings, such as those from wasp stings and other insect bites.

Its other use, in more longstanding circumstances, is to act as a diuretic and remove fluid from the body in some circulatory and respiratory conditions. It can also be used to promote urination when indicated.

Modalities: Better in the open air, cool bathing of the affected parts, and from moving about. Worse from any sort of heat, hot baths, stuffy rooms, from pressure and

24

lying down. Symptoms always appear worse around 5pm, on the right side, and after sleeping.

Suggested Potency: 30c.

Dosage: In acute situations, such as wasp stings, doses may be repeated every 10-15 minutes until the pain and swelling begin to subside. In other conditions a dose 3 to 4 times a day should be sufficient.

Additional Remedies: *Urtica* (see page 96) for irritable rashes rather than stings or bites.

Anecdote: Years ago, on television, I remember seeing a lady placing several bees onto the knee and elbow joints of patients, so that the stings would relieve arthritic pain.

When asked what the medical profession thought of such treatment, she replied, "they call me 'the bloody old quack from Bromley' but I don't mind if it helps people."

In homoeopathy, *Apis mel.* is indeed used as a treatment for some arthritic conditions. (FH)

APIS MEL.

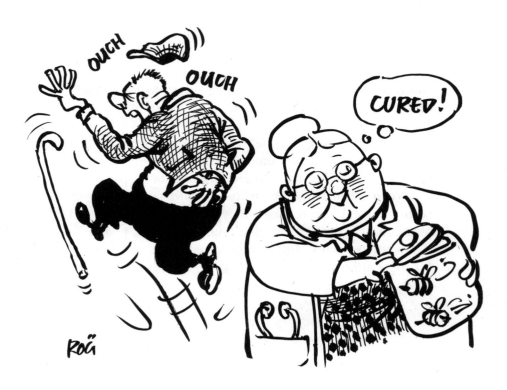

ARGENT. NIT. (Argentum nitricum)

Argent. nit., or silver nitrate, which is the English name for the substance, is a powerful caustic material and contact with it stains the skin black. Its use, in conventional medicine, had been as a 'styptic pencil' for controlling bleeding from small wounds and warts etc.

Argent. nit. has very different applications as a homoeopathic medicine. This remedy and *Gelsemium* (see page 60) are the two remedies that we consider, when 'fear' is the main symptom.

Keynotes: Anticipatory fear.

Uses:

1) For people and pets, to counteract anticipatory fears. These include exam nerves, public speaking, etc, for humans, and pre-show nerves for animals, especially in instances where contact with other animals may be a problem.

2) *Argent. nit.* is also a useful remedy for chronic eye conditions such as corneal opacity, with or without ulceration, and cataract.

3) It has a further use in treating gastric upsets where there is vomiting and watery, flatulent, diarrhoea, often accompanied by a marked feeling of bloating and distension of the abdomen (or stomach region). One particular symptom, that may help to lead to choosing this

remedy, is a craving for sweets and sweet things which then upset the patient further.

Modalities: Better for fresh air, and cold. Worse for warmth, stuffy rooms at night, and waking in the morning.

Suggested Potency: 6c or 30c.

Dosage: Pre-show, exam nerves etc, one tablet 3-4 times daily for 1 to 2 days before the event and one every 1 to 2 hours on the day itself. For other conditions, one dose 3 times daily for a few days as required.

Additional Remedies: *Gelsemium* (see page 60) for fear. *Euphrasia* (see page 58), *Silicea* (see page 86), and *Symphytum* (see page 93) for eye conditions. *Arsen. alb.* (see page 34) for vomiting and diarrhoea.

Anecdote: Soon after I attended a lecture at The Faculty of Homoeopathy in London, which included the uses of *Argent. nit.*, one of our nurses at the Practice told me she was about to take her driving test for the third time.

She was getting extremely nervous and very 'wound up', about the imminent test, and I persuaded her to try *Argent. nit.* as prescribed above.

Thankfully, she sailed through the driving test and, since then, the same remedy has helped others. It has also helped to calm numerous dogs before entering the Show Ring. (FH)

ARGENT NIT.

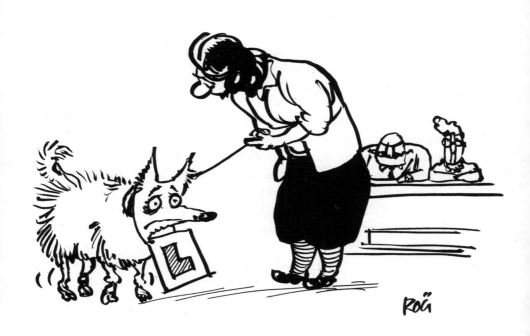

ARNICA (Arnica montana)

Arnica is a member of the large family of plants known as the Compositae (the daisy family) and grows at high altitudes. It has been well known for centuries as a valuable topical application for injuries and bruising. It grows freely on the mountains in Switzerland and is used there to relieve the pain and discomfort of knocks and bruises etc, sustained whilst skiing.

Arnica must be amongst the best known of all homoeopathic remedies and many, who know nothing about homoeopathy, have heard of it.

When we talk to various groups of people around the country about homoeopathy, we usually finish by trying to persuade them to get some *Arnica* tablets, if nothing else, and keep them in the house. They will inevitably come in useful for treating all those minor household accidents that cause bruising and discomfort.

Arnica may follow the use of *Aconite* (see page 21), or itself be used as a first remedy, to be followed in turn by another selected remedy, according to the condition being treated. Homoeopathy is all about matching the symptoms, presented, as accurately as possible with the appropriate remedy. If this can be achieved, the results can be spectacular but disappointment can also result, if the wrong remedy is chosen. *Arnica* has done more than anything else to convert people to homoeopathy.

Keynotes: Bruising, inflammation.

Uses: For any ailment or condition which involves inflammation, bruising, stiffness, soreness and/or bleeding. *Arnica* possesses the most wonderful healing properties and can even prevent a thing like a 'black eye' developing, if it is administered soon enough. It is also most useful before and after operations of any sort (minor or major) and before and after dental treatment. It can also be used for mental and physical exhaustion.

Modalities: Worse for touch and movement. Better when lying down.

Suggested Potency: 6c or 30c. I prefer to use *Arnica* in a 30c potency but, either in a 6c or a 30c, it should give beneficial results.

Dosage: As a first aid treatment, *Arnica* may be usefully given every $1/2 - 1$ hour, according to the severity of the condition, for up to 6 doses and then 3 to 4 times daily, as necessary. It should be taken **prior** to surgery for 3-5 days, at the acute level (3-4 times daily).

Additional Remedies: *Aconite* (see page 21) for shock. *Rhus tox.* (see page 83) after injuries. *Hypericum* (see page 67) for pain. *Bellis* (see page 99), the daisy, is also useful for some types of injuries with much soreness; it is claimed that *Bellis* is especially effective when injury, or trauma, to the breast is involved.

Anecdotes:

1) Expectant mothers often appear at the Surgery with their pets, for treatment, and I always make a point of extolling the virtues of homoeopathy in general and *Arnica* in particular before, during, and after childbirth.

Quite often the client leaves with some treatment for their animal, plus a vial of *Arnica* tablets and some relevant literature for themselves! (FH)

2) Of all the thousand or so remedies in common use, *Arnica* is one of our best 'advertising agents' for homoeopathy because it never fails to perform.

My elder son was a keen rugby player in his early days. Following a season of playing and training hard, he was invited to attend an international students' trial. After days of anticipation, we drove for six hours to reach the venue and, within 30 seconds of the kick-off, son number one had collided with an 18 stone monster in his own team!   He was carried off dazed but not concussed.

After 6 doses of *Arnica*, at 5 minute intervals, he was well enough to return to the game and, indeed, secured his place in the final squad. (SK)

3) The value of *Arnica*, prior to dental surgery, was illustrated by the following case.

Many years ago, my wife needed to have her wisdom teeth extracted. The right side of her mouth was dealt with first. She was in a terrible state, having to spend a day in bed and suffering from a tender mouth for many days afterwards.

But before having the left tooth out, she took *Arnica* 30c tablets, 3 times daily, for 3 days, and then every 10 minutes for 6 doses, immediately after the extraction.

She was well enough to go to a dance, the same night, with minimal discomfort. (SK)

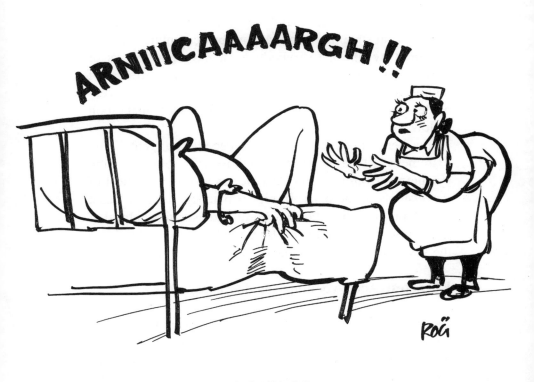

ARNICA

ARSEN. ALB. (Arsenicum album)

Arsenicum album or white arsenic (arsenious oxide), as it is commonly called, is a very emotive substance. Its poisonous properties are well known and, in real life and in fiction down the ages, it has been involved in many cases of criminal poisoning.

This is another prime example of Dr Samuel Hahnemann's maxim 'Similia similibus curentur' ('let like be cured by like'). Everybody must have read books or newspaper articles describing the striking effects of administering quite small amounts of Arsenic, and the very acute symptoms of vomiting and diarrhoea that soon follow.

In homoeopathic potency, it becomes a gentle and extremely fast acting antidote to those very same dramatic symptoms. Homoeopathic Arsenic has an effect on most of the systems of the body. In higher potency, it can act as a stimulant to both mind and body and is often helpful if given in cases of terminal disease, when it is said to have the same effect as a Gin and Tonic!

Keynotes: Acute vomiting and diarrhoea.

Uses: Food poisoning of any sort, bacterial or toxin induced, will almost always benefit from a few doses of *Arsen. alb.* Its many other uses include conjunctivitis, allergies, hay fever, some forms of asthma, loss of appetite,

34

parvovirus infection in dogs, and various types of skin condition such as eczema and scurf (dandruff).

Modalities: Worse in wet weather, and after midnight, and from cold of any sort - air, draughts, food, or drink. Better for heat, sitting up, and warm drinks.

Suggested Potency: 6c or 30c.

Dosage:

1) Acute: Every 10-20 minutes up to 6 doses, if required, then 4 times daily for 2-3 days as necessary.

2) Chronic: a dose 4 times daily, for up to 7 days, should be sufficient: if not, a different remedy may be required. If symptoms persist, particularly in cases of chronic diarrhoea, professional help should be sought.

Additional Remedies: *Merc. sol.* (see page 70) and *Podophyllum* (see page 76) for diarrhoea without vomiting.

Anecdote: One of the first animals that I treated with this excellent remedy was Ben, an 8-week-old Labrador puppy, with hyper-acute vomiting (being sick every 5-10 minutes) and, by the time I examined him, there was really nothing left to bring up.

After half a dozen doses of *Arsen. alb.* at 10 minute intervals, the vomiting had ceased and a very 'sorry' puppy was once again bouncing about and driving its owner mad!

I make a point of never telling the owner, until after their beloved pet is better again, that I am prescribing Arsenic. The average owner cannot handle this piece of information until improvement is complete! (FH)

ARSEN. ALB.

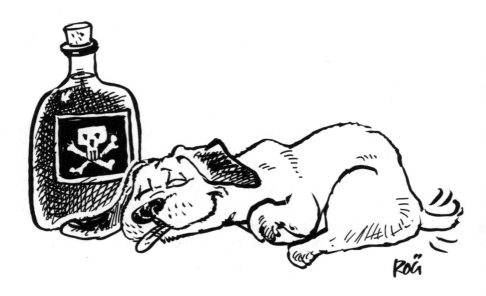

BELLADONNA (Atropa belladonna)

This plant grows in many European countries, is commonly known as 'deadly nightshade' and it is a member of the family Solanaceae. This family also contains the red peppers (Capsicum), tobacco (Nicotiana tabacum), and another useful homoeopathic remedy, *Dulcamara* (bittersweet), which is also very poisonous but again, homoeopathically, makes a powerful medicine.

'Bella donna' (beautiful lady) gets its name from about 500 years ago, when Italian ladies used to put the juice in their eyes to enlarge the pupils and thereby make their eyes look larger, darker, shining, and, consequently, their faces more beautiful. The berries are big, juicy, and black and not unlike cherries to look at. They taste very sweet which makes them potentially extremely dangerous, especially to children.

Belladonna has a profound effect on the nervous and vascular (heart and circulation) systems. Symptoms are usually rapid in onset, severe, and even violent at times.

Keynotes: Acute fever and high temperature. Bad temper. Aggression.

Uses: Any sort of fever accompanied by high temperature, rapid bounding pulse, throbbing head and dilated pupils should respond to *Belladonna*. One feature that often indicates the remedy is an extremely sudden onset of symptoms. *Belladonna* can be used to alleviate the dramatic and distressing symptoms of heatstroke and, also, may help control many types of fits. Finally, it is beneficial in controlling aggression in groups of animals.

Modalities: Worse for bright light, noise of any sort, and jolting or jarring. Symptoms are worse around 3pm. Better for warmth, rest, and as little movement as possible.

Suggested Potency: 30c.

Dosage: Initially, doses every 30-60 minutes for up to 6 or 8 doses may be required. In very acute fevers, the frequency can be increased to every 15 minutes. Subsequently, one dose every 4 hours for a few days, according to response.

Additional Remedies: *Staphysagria*, (see page 101) for resentment, and *Lachesis*, (see page 100) for jealousy, could also be considered in this context. For instance, if a new pet is introduced to the household, and there is friction or difficulty in getting them to settle down together.

Anecdote: "Catflap Charlie" or "CC", as he was known, was a large, roundheaded, fierce, ginger cat and he had been 'doctored' when he was fully grown. During the early part of his life he had been a stray, fending for himself.

When he finally decided to settle down, he adopted a household which contained four other cats. The owners soon found out that they lived in "CC's" house, rather than the other way round, which often seems to be the case in homes that have cats! "CC" guarded the cat-flap and terrorised the other cats, who did not dare to come in or out when he was around. A dose of *Belladonna*, given once or twice a week for 6 weeks, sorted "CC" out.

He then became friendly to his house-mates and affectionate to his owners. (FH)

BELLADONNA

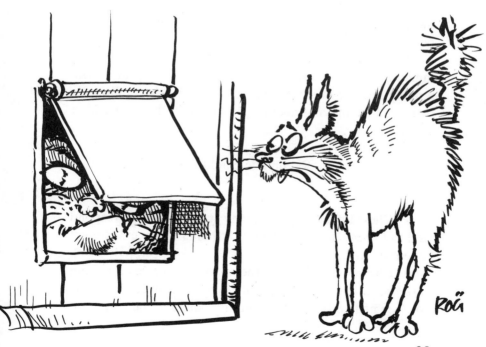

BRYONIA (Bryonia alba)

There are about twenty varieties of Bryonia growing in different countries around the world. Bryonia belongs to the Cucurbitaceae (the gourd or pumpkin family) which also contains another useful remedy, *Colocynthis*. Common names for the plant are white bryony or wild hops. One of these, Bryonia dioica, is found in Britain but the one used in homoeopathic medicine is *Bryonia alba* and this grows in Europe. It is a climbing hedgerow plant with a massive twisted white root from which the mother tincture is prepared. It is said that, in the past, the white root, which is poisonous, was sold as a substitute for the more exotic mandrake root, reputed from biblical times to be a potent aphrodisiac.

The phrase 'worse for movement' sums up the indications when this remedy could be helpful. The remedy may be useful whenever the patient's condition is worsened by moving about. This is often the case with a cough.

Keynotes: Cough. Rheumatic conditions. Toothache.

Uses:

1) Chest infections, and many types of cough, respond well to *Bryonia* and it is useful for flu in people and 'kennel cough' in dogs.

2) Chronic arthritis and rheumatism often benefit from *Bryonia*. Sometimes, the remedy is followed by *Rhus tox.* (see page 83) if the symptoms change to indicate it or,

40

if the symptom picture is not too clear, the remedies may be alternated once or twice daily.

3) Mastitis, inflammation of the mammary glands (or breasts), particularly if there is more pain when even slight pressure is applied.

4) Toothache. The ache seems to go from tooth to tooth and can extend to the cheeks or the whole head, becoming a headache.

5) Nosebleeds, especially before a period is due.

Modalities: Worse for warmth and any movement. Worse in hot weather, in the morning, and from the least touch or exertion. Better in a cold atmosphere, from cold drinks, from rest, from lying on the affected side, and from pressure.

Suggested Potency: 6c.

Dosage: 4-6 times daily, reducing the frequency as the condition improves.

Additional Remedies: *Rhus tox.* (see page 83).

Anecdote: Zebedee, the aged donkey, had a great similarity in appearance to Eeyore in A.A.Milne's "Winnie the Pooh". He seemed to 'sag', was very dejected, creaking and coughing with every faltering step he took and his poor old nose dripped constantly. Needless to say, he appeared to be both sad and depressed.

Bryonia given 4 times daily on a small piece of toast, for a week, improved him enormously. Thereafter, *Bryonia* was given 2-3 times daily whenever the cough or stiffness returned. (FH)

BRYONIA

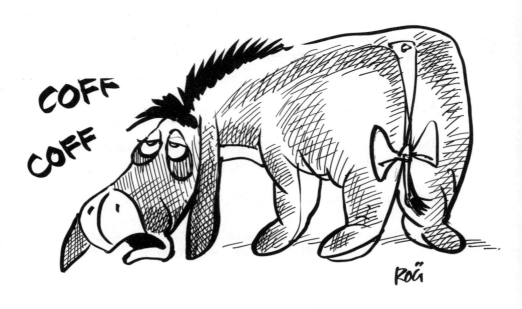

CANTHARIS (Spanish Fly)

The remedy is initially prepared by trituration (see page 6) of the entire insect, also sometimes known as the blister beetle, and subsequently mixing it in alcohol and making the various potencies.

This remedy should always be considered when there is acute burning pain, especially in the bladder and the region of the kidneys. Spanish Fly has been used for many years, in its natural state, as an aphrodisiac and with disastrous results.

Keynotes: Sudden onset. Burning pains. Blister formation.

Uses:

1) The most important use of this remedy is in the treatment and relief of the pain caused by acute cystitis. Antibiotics may well be needed at the outset but *Cantharis*, given at the same time, will certainly help to relieve the acute pain and discomfort. In chronic recurring cases, *Cantharis* is also useful and, in this instance, antibiotics may not be necessary. A short course of *Cantharis,* given for 3-5 days monthly, may well prevent attacks of cystitis occurring so frequently.

2) Blisters and vesicles on the skin, accompanied by intense irritation, respond well to *Cantharis*.

3) Acute burns, scalds, insect bites and mouth ulcers may all be treated with *Cantharis*

Modalities: Worse from touch, drinking cold water or coffee, and passing water when suffering from cystitis. Better for warmth, and rubbing the sore place.

Suggested Potency: 6c and 30c can both be useful.

Dosage: In the first aid situation, a dose may be given every 15-20 minutes up to 4 times, followed by doses at 2-4 hourly intervals for 4 to 7 days.

Additional Remedies: *Apis mel*. (see page 24) and *Urtica* (see page 96).

Anecdote: Jenny, the miniature Dachshund, suffered from frequent bouts of cystitis, especially in cold and wet weather.

Jenny's small body was carried very near to the ground and this may well have contributed to the attacks because, when Jenny squatted, she actually touched the ground and could easily get 'chilled'.

Routine courses of *Cantharis* given every month, or more often if required, helped to control this condition. (FH)

CANTHARIS

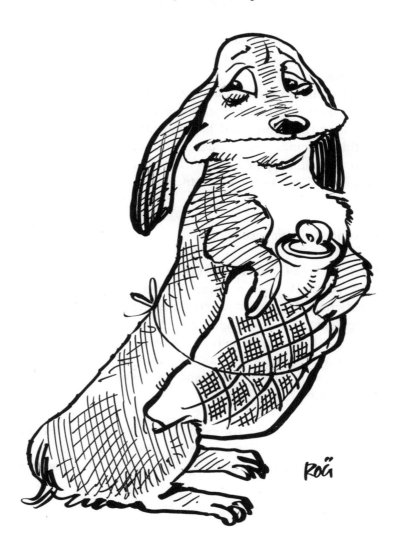

CARBO VEG. (Carbo vegetabilis)

Black charcoal is the basis of this remedy. It may be prepared by heating any kind of wood to 'red heat' to burn off the gases, and the ash (charcoal) is then made into the remedy *Carbo veg.* Today, *Carbo veg.* is made from the birch tree.

Charcoal, in its natural state, is an inert substance but, like two other remedies *Lycopodium* and *Silicea* which are also inert, once prepared homoeopathically they become useful medicines. The powdered charcoal is prepared to the third centesimal potency by trituration (see page 6) and then diluted and succussed in the normal manner (see page 6-9).

Keynotes: Flatulence. Collapse.

Uses: Where flatulence occurs, particularly in some dogs (and people!) after a meal, *Carbo veg.* can be very beneficial. Because of its power to act on the circulatory system, in cases of collapse, it is sometimes affectionately known as "the corpse reviver". *Carbo veg.* can be helpful in controlling halitosis (bad breath), mouth ulcers, and sneezing with running eyes and nose which may, in turn, lead to chronic nose bleeding.

Modalities: Worse for cold, frosty weather, open air, evening and night. A hot stuffy atmosphere and humid conditions also make matters worse. Both these sets of conditions can intensify the lack of oxygen. Somewhat better for vigorous fanning and belching.

Suggested Potency: 6c for flatulence etc, 30c for collapse.

Dosage: For flatulence, it is advisable to adjust the dose to obtain the best results. As a guide, a tablet given an hour before and another an hour after eating is often sufficient, but more frequent dosing may be necessary. In cases of sudden collapse, a tablet may be placed under the tongue, or powdered and tipped into the mouth, every 10-15 minutes up to 4-6 times if required, while professional help is being sought. For other conditions, a dose given 3-4 times daily, for a few days, should suffice.

Additional Remedies: *Nux vomica* (see page 73) for digestive upsets. *Aconite* (see page 21) and *Arnica* (see page 30) for shock and collapse.

Anecdote: Cicero, the Great Dane, was very unsocial and frequently passed extremely offensive odours, which often necessitated opening the windows or even vacating the room for a while!

Dosing with *Carbo veg.*, once or twice daily, did the trick nicely and controlled this unfortunate habit. (FH)

CARBO VEG.

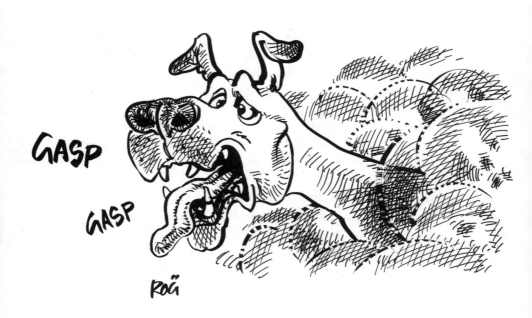

CHAMOMILLA (Matricaria chamomilla)

Chamomilla is a member of the family Compositae (the daisy family) and its common name is wild chamomile. It is interesting that this little wild flower demonstrates its remedy properties in its manner of growth. The plant grows very rapidly with great energy and determination and the shoot, leaf, and flower spring up together, becoming fully formed within two months. This enables the plant to produce two crops in a season.

Many may remember the television play "The Camomile Lawn" and, today, herbal tea is still made from chamomile to help relieve indigestion and to overcome insomnia.

Wild chamomile, by its manner of growth and development, suggests a rapid, perhaps exaggerated, reaction to events and impatience is paramount.

Keynotes: Frantic pain. Rage. Teething.

Uses: Extreme pain which, to the patient concerned, is often intolerable, to a degree far worse than the illness or condition might suggest. Toothache can usually be controlled by *Chamomilla*. It is also useful in controlling rage in babies and young children. Any pain which makes the patient extremely restless, moving about almost in a frenzy at times, points towards the remedy *Chamomilla*.

Modalities: Worse for being hot or angry, and in the open air. Better for warm, humid and wet weather. Babies get comfort from being carried, or travelling in a car.

Suggested Potency: 30c.

Dosage: Every 10-15 minutes, up to 6 doses, and then continue, for acute cases, 3-4 times daily for a day or two, as required.

Additional Remedies: *Aconite* (see page 21). *Arnica* (see page 30). *Cantharis* (see page 43). *Hypericum* (see page 67).

Anecdotes:

1) At dinner with friends one night, the 4-month-old baby suddenly woke up screaming and very peevish. The mother brought Angela downstairs and she had a bright red blob on one cheek and was obviously 'teething' and in distress. A little *Chamomilla* powder was placed on her tongue, and the dose repeated after 10 minutes, and Angela was soon peacefully asleep again. So it was that the Vet was able to relieve the baby's toothache! (FH)

2) My partner's 10-month-old baby used to lie on the floor having a tantrum, screaming and kicking furiously with his legs. Fortunately, it was always possible to get a little *Chamomilla* into his mouth and he, very soon, calmed down. (FH)

3) Coming back from a visit to the USA recently, I and all my fellow passengers were kept awake by a child screaming for what seemed like **hours**. The mother was exasperated, explaining in a loud voice that it was teething and had colic.

Fortunately, I had my travelling pack of remedies and offered the mother some *Chamomilla*. She was a little unsure, at first, but, when the baby quietened down, after only two doses, her fear evaporated! When we finally reached our destination, several appreciative passengers enquired as to what had been administered. (SK)

CHAMOMILLA

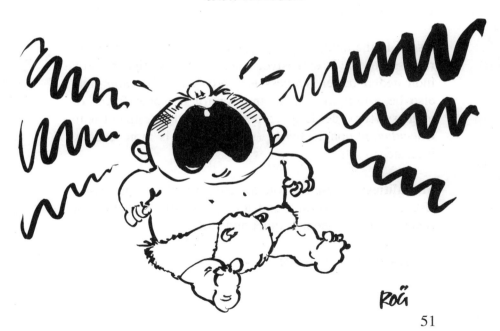

Roü

51

COCCULUS (Cocculus indicus)

Cocculus indicus is the name given to the seed of the plant Anamirta cocculus which grows along the coast in parts of India and Ceylon. It belongs to the plant family Menispermaceae and is more commonly known as the indian cockle. *Cocculus* contains the powerful poison, Picrotoxin, which has a 'drugging' effect and was formerly used to enhance the intoxicating properties of cheap beer and porter.

In the older homoeopathic books, its use is recommended for "the ill effects of travelling in a carriage".

Keynotes: Vertigo. Nausea.

Uses: In the modern world where travel, whether by road, rail, sea or air is extensive, *Cocculus* is the first remedy indicated if travel sickness is a problem. *Cocculus* may also be useful to help in the control of some forms of epilepsy (fits). Jet Lag can respond well to treatment with *Cocculus*, although *Arnica* (see page 30) is more usually indicated.

Modalities: Worse for cold air and open air. From loss of sleep, eating, travelling and jolting or jarring. Better for lying down and keeping quiet and still.

Suggested Potency: 30c.

Dosage: One dose to be given about 45-60 minutes before travelling, followed by a second dose just before starting the journey. The dose may be repeated, every hour or so, if required but it may be found that just a single dose, given a little while before starting out, is sufficient.

Additional Remedies: In the cases where *Cocculus* does not prove to be effective in the control of travel or motion sickness, the remedies *Nux vomica* (see page 73), *Petroleum* (see page 101) and *Tabacum* (see page 101) may also be considered, especially if a sea journey is involved.

In addition to administering a remedy, other measures can be taken to reduce discomfort to pets. Allowing the animal to sit on the floor of the vehicle, frequent stops, and availability of water to drink, are all important.

Anecdote: Mrs Green asked me, one day, if there was a good remedy for travel sickness for her Labrador dog, Trampus. I naturally prescribed *Cocculus* to be given as indicated above.

Several months later, I met Mrs Green again and asked how Trampus was reacting to the *Cocculus*. The reply was as follows: "Oh! I haven't had to use it for Trampus yet, but I take a dose myself before I go on a long car journey and it stops me feeling ill and helps me to keep alert. It also helped to prevent air sickness on a holiday flight recently!" (FH)

COCCULUS

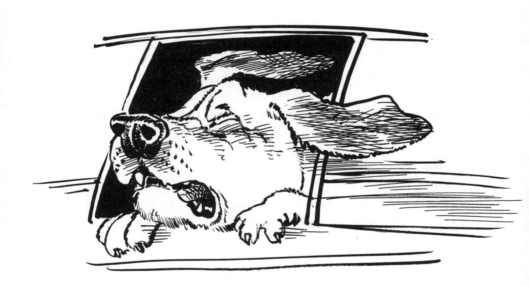

ROČI

COLOCYNTHIS (Cucumis colocynthis)

Colocynthis, whose common name is bitter (or squirting) cucumber, is a member of the plant family Cucurbitaceae. The family also contains pumpkins and gourds, and the fruit of the colocynthis plant looks something like an orange, in size and colour. It is an interesting fact that, with homoeopathy, the habits of a number of plants are reflected in the symptoms displayed by the patient. In the case of *Colocynthis*, the plant grows in a twisting and twining fashion which rather resembles the writhing and contortions of a patient with acute colic or 'collywobbles'.

The first three letters 'Col' of *Colocynthis* at once puts us in mind of colic, which makes an easy way to remember the principal action of this remedy.

In ancient times it was used in Eastern countries, in its herbal state, as a purgative and also to induce abortion, and its main habitat is the eastern Mediterranean.

Keynotes: Acute abdominal pain. Sudden onset. Unable to keep still during spasms.

Uses: This is the first remedy to consider in cases of sudden and violent abdominal pain. Colic may occur in most animals and, of course, is quite frequently seen in young babies, as well as older people.

A most spectacular form of colic can, unfortunately, affect horses who may get up and down constantly, throw themselves about, roll backwards and forwards, and even die from a twisted bowel.

Modalities: Worse for cold wind and damp, eating raw fruit, iced drinks etc. Also worse from rage, or anger, from indignation. Better for warmth, firm pressure, bending double, and applying local heat.

Suggested Potency: 30c.

Dosage: One tablet every 5-15 minutes, up to 6 doses if necessary, followed by a dose every hour until the symptoms and pain are relieved. All the remedies are available in powder form so it is easy, and perfectly safe, to put a little powder (it does not have to be the whole powder) on a baby's tongue if it shows signs of colic.
   CAUTION: If colic symptoms persist, or worsen, it is important to seek medical or veterinary assistance immediately.

Additional Remedies: *Chamomilla* (see page 49) for toothache and pains during teething. *Nux Vomica* (see page 73) for the pains of over indulgence (in the head or in the stomach, i.e. a hangover!). *Cocculus* (see page 52) for discomfort or pains while travelling.

Anecdote: The first time he had colic, Donald the donkey was 23 years old. It was Christmas Day, and the Vet had to be sent for as an emergency. The owner was advised to keep some *Colcynthis* in hand, in case of further troubles. Once again, on Christmas Day, Donald showed signs of mild colic developing which responded, immediately, to a few doses of *Colocynthis*.

Why did Donald get colic on Christmas Day? The reason turned out to be that Donald attended the Nativity Service, in the local church, on Christmas Day and over-indulged on lots of tit-bits and mints, given to him by the children, at the end of the service. (FH)

COLOCYNTHIS

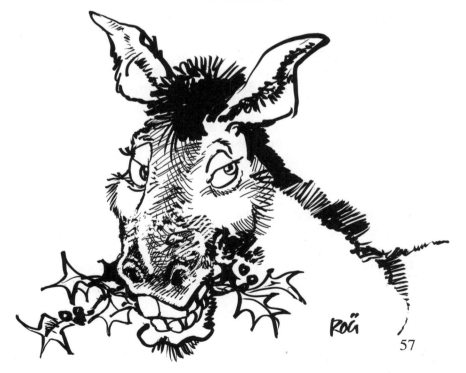

EUPHRASIA (Euphrasia officinalis)

Euphrasia is also known as 'eyebright' and belongs to the plant family Scrophulariaceas. The name 'eyebright' given to this plant, since early times, is interesting because it neatly describes its action.

We have included this remedy simply because of its very beneficial action in many eye conditions. It acts on the mucous membrane (the tissue) surrounding the eye which, if it becomes inflamed, causes extra production of tears. *Euphrasia* also acts on the front surface of the eye itself (the cornea).

Keynotes: Sore eyes.

Uses: The treatment of conjunctivitis, which often becomes chronic and persistent. *Euphrasia* can also be used beneficially to treat damage to the cornea, caused by ulceration.

Modalities: Better from cold water. Sore eyes are said to be helped by drinking coffee. Worse from sunlight and rubbing the eyes.

Suggested Potency: Diluted mother tincture for local administration (see below). 30c when taken by mouth.

Dosage: This is the only remedy in this book which is used in its original form as a mother tincture. ONE drop only of mother tincture is placed in a half pint mug of freshly boiled and cooled water or sterile water. The resulting solution is then used in an eye bath or, for animals, as an eye wash. It is important not to have this eye wash too strong or it can irritate the eyes. Therefore, if two drops come out of the stock bottle, empty half the liquid away and top up with more boiled or sterile water. *Euphrasia* may also be taken, in tablet form, to supplement the action of the local application.

CAUTION: Any eye condition is potentially serious so it is important to seek professional help, sooner rather than later. It is, however, quite safe to use *Euphrasia* eye wash in conjunction with antibiotics, etc. **Do not use the Euphrasia 'mother tincture' undiluted.**

Anecdote: Blanche, as her name implied, was a white and a very beautiful and well groomed miniature poodle. Unfortunately, Blanche suffered from permanently discharging eyes and the acrid tears caused an unsightly brown streak running down from the inner corner of both eyes. Thanks to the frequent use of *Euphrasia*, this condition improved enormously. (FH)

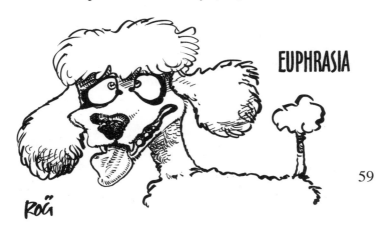

EUPHRASIA

GELSEMIUM (Gelsemium sempervirens)

Yellow jasmine, as it is commonly known, grows in North America. It is a member of the Loganaceae family and so is not, in fact, a true jasmine at all. This family also includes buddleias with their lovely scent and fascinating attraction for butterflies.

Gelsemium contains two principle alkaloids, both of which are very poisonous. Gelseminine, one of the two, has an action rather like Strychnine - causing rigidity and paralysis. However, once it has been prepared into a homoeopathic medicine, it is perfectly safe and has several uses.

Its main action is upon the body's nervous system and it should be considered where virus infections, with possibly toxic effects, are involved. Orthodox medicine does not have a lot to offer when viruses are implicated, and this is when homoeopathy can be so helpful and effective.

Keynotes: Fear and influenza (see below).

Uses: Many kinds of flu, in people of all ages, and also as an additional treatment in cases of equine- and cat-flu. There is great heaviness and tiredness of body and limbs with aches and pains all over. The other important characteristic of *Gelsemium* is its action when fear is present or anticipated. 'Shaking with fright' and shivering (as in flu) point to *Gelsemium*.

Modalities: Worse for damp weather, fog, and thunderstorms, being in a hot room, and from excitement. Better in open air and moving about, if the effort can be made; also from stimulants.

Suggested Potency: 30c.

Dosage: For FLU: see below.
          For FEAR: Dose hourly for 3-4 hours, before the event which is causing the concern.

Additional Remedies: Compare *Argent. nit.* (see page 27). Also *Borax* (see page 99) for fear of loud noises, such as thunder, and fireworks on bonfire night etc.

For influenza:
There are a number of useful flu remedies in the homoeopathic armoury and it is important, as with choosing any remedy, to match the symptoms as nearly as possible to the remedy picture.

> *Gelsemium* - sneezing, cold and hot alternately, shivering, and aches and pains all over.
> *Arsenicum album* - with streaming eyes and nose, and chilliness.
> *Baptisia* - with high fever and gastric symptoms.
> *Bryonia* - with great thirst for cold fluids and a cough, causing headache.
> *Eupatorium perfoliatum* - with bursting headache, shivering, and aching in limbs and back.

Nux vomica - with stomach upset, and chilliness.
Pyrogenium -with very rapid pulse and intense restlessness.

Dosage: One tablet every 2 hours, up to 8 times, on the first day, then 4 times daily (every 4 hours) for the next 3-5 days, as long as symptoms persist.

Anecdote: One of the advantages of using homoeopathic remedies with veterinary patients is that they do not affect normal animal functions in the same way that conventional medicines might.

For example, a homoeopathic remedy such as *Cocculus* (see page 52) may be given for motion sickness, but this will not sedate the animal completely for an hour or two after the journey has ended.

One particular example of this can be related. Some years ago, a lady came to my pharmacy requesting some *Gelsemium* for her Sheltie bitch. This breed is particularly apt to become excitable and anxious, especially when strangers are about. *Gelsemium* works well in this situation and so I dispensed the remedy, as requested.

About three days later, the lady returned with her hand heavily bandaged. I enquired, "whatever happened to you?" "Well," she said, "the *Gelsemium* seemed to be working so well, and the dog had quietened down so much, that I thought I would test your idea about the the animal's natural instincts not being affected. I tried to take her feeding bowl away from her while she was eating." "And?" I said, in expectation! "The dashed thing bit me", she cried. (SK)

GELSEMIUM

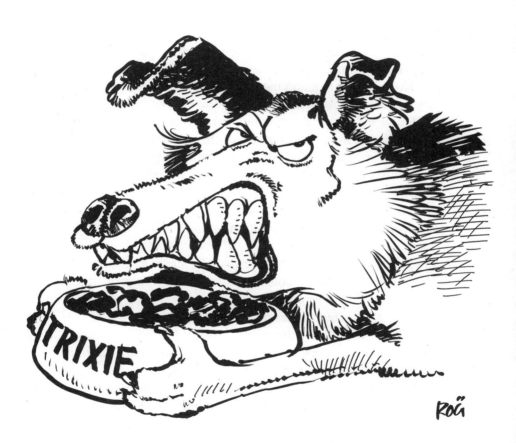

HEPAR SULPH. (Hepar sulphuris calcareum)

Hepar sulph. is a rather fascinating remedy in that it was developed by Dr Hahnemann himself. The medicine is prepared from equal parts of finely ground oyster shells and pure Flowers of Sulphur. These are heated to 'white heat' and kept at this temperature for ten minutes. The remedy is prepared from the ash that forms.

How Dr Hahnemann came to make this remedy, in the first place, is not clear. It is clear, however, that it has a profound effect on the mucous membranes of the body. These are the lining membranes of the different systems of the body, such as the digestive and respiratory systems.

It also has a beneficial effect on the skin when it becomes infected.

Keynotes: Infection. Suppuration.

Uses: All types of infection, especially chronic infection. *Hepar sulph.* could be considered to be the homoeopathic equivalent of an antibiotic because its action is principally directed at infected tissues and glands.

Hepar sulph. is, therefore, useful to treat various conditions in the eyes, ears and chest, and skin, particularly where sepsis and pus formation are present.

CAUTION: Infections, particularly in young children, such as earache, may well need antibiotics and this fact should not be overlooked. However, it is safe and often advantageous, especially in repeated episodes of infection, to use antibiotics and *Hepar sulph.* together, or following one another.

Modalities: Worse from cold, dry winds, draughts or cool air. Particularly susceptible to slight touch or pressure from which the pain can seem intolerable. Better for warmth and warm, damp, weather.

Suggested Potency: 30c.

Dosage: A dose, 3-4 times daily, for a few days (3 to 5 days is usually sufficient). This may be repeated, after a week, if necessary. In chronic infections, such as those that commonly occur in the ears and in the anal glands of dogs, periodic treatment, for a few days each month, may be required to keep a chronic infection in check.

Additional Remedies: *Sulphur* (see page 90) in chronic infections, particularly when the skin is involved. *Silicea* (see page 86) is another remedy to consider in chronic conditions.

Anecdote: Bodger was an enormous ginger cat, of uncertain age, and he had been 'doctored' rather later in life.
   When he finally settled down in the new home, that he decided to adopt, he began to display unsocial tendencies! Bodger, all his life, had enjoyed a fight and as he got older, and less nimble, he was always getting bitten and developing abscesses.

As time went by, these became more and more difficult to clear up with antibiotics and he would come to the surgery with one side of his face badly swollen, almost as if he had mumps! Regular courses of *Hepar sulph.* helped to keep these chronic infections under control. (FH)

HEPAR SULPH.

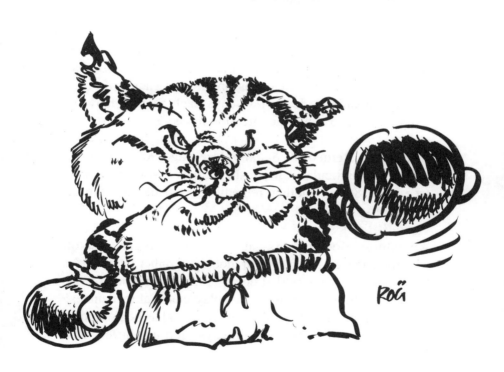

HYPERICUM (Hypericum perforatum)

This remedy is prepared from the wild plant, St John's wort, which grows in abundance in open woods and along hedge banks. Since the Middle Ages, its beneficial properties in helping to heal wounds have been known. In those days, St John's wort was also thought to have the power to repel witches and the doings of evil spirits (wizards etc).

The mother tincture is made from the whole fresh plant and is used externally, as well as being potentised (see page 7) and taken by mouth.

Keynotes: Wounds. Pain.

Uses: It has a particularly soothing effect in torn or lacerated wounds, when nerve endings have been damaged. *Hypericum* is also useful in treating burns and scalds.

Hypericum is combined with *Calendula* (Marigold) to produce a soothing and healing ointment or cream, known as HyperCal® cream (see page 103). It can also be combined with the remedy *Cantharis* (see page 43) to form an external application which, if applied immediately after a burn or scald, can be just as effective as a medication containing steroids (cortisone).

When given internally, it helps to control many sorts of pain, particularly in the lower back, and also if fingers, toes, and nails become crushed. Pain after operations can also be eased by taking *Hypericum*.

Modalities: Worse in cold air and damp weather, if foggy, and from touch and movement. Worse also between 6pm and 10pm, and in the dark. Better from keeping still, and bending the head backwards.

Suggested Potency: 30c.

Dosage: *Hypericum*, by mouth, should be taken every 2-4 hours initially and then 3-4 times daily, for as long as required. The ointments and creams come prepared, ready for use, and may be applied several times daily (see page 102).

Additional Remedies: *Ledum palustre* (marsh tea) (see page 100) is another valuable remedy for treating wounds, especially puncture wounds and animal bites. *Arnica* (see page 30) should also be kept in mind, where injuries with inflammation and bruising have occurred, and may well be used before *Hypericum* or *Ledum*.

Anecdotes:

1) *Hypericum* is often called "the blood and crush" remedy. The Hypericum bush has a charming yellow flower which, when crushed, becomes red rather like blood.

My wife and I had returned to our home airport, after a long transatlantic flight, and we were waiting for our baggage when I noticed a small boy playing on the carousel. To my horror, he decided to try to retrieve a sweet just as the carousel was switched on. He screamed with pain as his finger was crushed. Luckily I had a vial of *Hypericum* granules in my pocket and, with the mother's permission, I administered some granules every five minutes until the ambulance arrived. The boy's discomfort appeared to subside quickly.

Homoeopathic remedies can be given safely in the knowledge that they will not interfere with any subsequent or concurrent treatment. I also gave the mother *Aconite* for shock! (SK)

2) An interesting property of the remedy *Hypericum* is that it may be associated with people who like wine. You can imagine my amusement, therefore, when the President of the local Wine Club came in for advice, having shut his finger in the lid of a wooden crate! (SK)

HYPERICUM

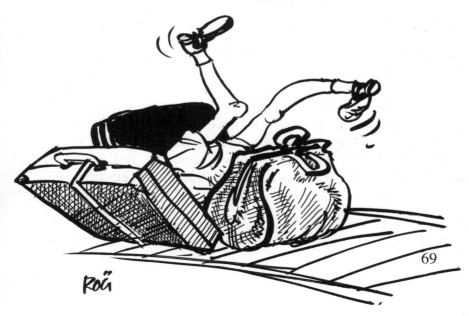

Roü

MERC. SOL. (Mercurius solubilis)

Mercury, as a homoeopathic medicine, was introduced by Hahnemann himself in 1778. It was prepared using the trituration method (see page 6) from the element liquid mercury. Mercury is another example of Dr Hahnemann's diligent research to find new and very varying substances with widely differing actions to prepare his remedies.

Mercury is also known as Quicksilver. This is the silver liquid which spills from the thermometer when you drop it or knock it against something at the critical moment when you need it most!

Mercury, in its natural state, has a profound poisoning effect on a number of the systems and tissues of the body. Mercury affects the mouth, giving it a metallic taste, and the production of large amounts of saliva. It also inflames the throat, stomach, and bowel and, on excretion, damages the kidneys causing nephritis. In addition, the poison can be secreted through the skin.

Keynotes: Acute enteritis (diarrhoea). Acute skin problems.

Uses: For acute otitis in children and animals, where the discharge is copious and may smell offensive. Likewise, offensive breath and inflamed gums (gingivitis) respond to *Merc. sol.* Diarrhoea alone, without vomiting, and acute wet eczema are two other conditions that will benefit from *Merc. sol.*

Modalities: Worse from extremes of weather, particularly worse at night. Worse, when perspiring in a warm room or bed and when lying on the right side. Better, but only slightly, when resting.

Suggested Potency: 6c or 30c.

Dosage: Initially one dose every 2 hours, up to 6 times on the first day, then 4 times daily, for 4-7 days, as required.

Additional Remedies: *Arsen. alb.* (see page 34), when both vomiting and diarrhoea occur simultaneously. *Merc. corr.* (see page 100) when diarrhoea leads to persistent straining or when any of the conditions mentioned above are very intense. *Podophyllum* (see page 76) is another useful diarrhoea remedy.

Anecdote: Ben, a young Labrador, was put in the kennels for a couple of days while his owners took a well-earned weekend break from him.

Ben was lovely, but very naughty, and had chewed up clothes, curtains and some of the children's toys, to say nothing of gnawing chair legs and stair rods etc!

Ben developed wet eczema, while he was in the kennels, probably, in part at least, due to the stress of being separated from his loved ones for the first time. Large patches of wet, sticky eczema (as big as a saucer) can occur in minutes, with the combination of the intense irritation and continual licking.

Ben was treated, at once, in the kennels with repeated doses of *Merc. sol.* and the lesion soon dried up and was forgotten. He was content in the kennels but, Oh! what joy for all when his folks returned and they were all together again. (FH)

MERC. SOL.

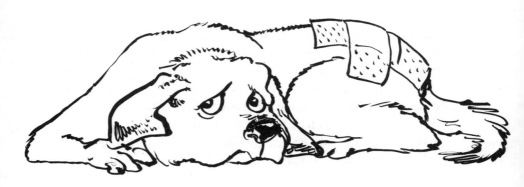

NUX VOMICA (Strychnos nux vomica)

Nux vomica, known as the poison nut, comes from a tree that grows in the East Indies, Northern Australia and Malaysia. The tree belongs to the order Loganiacea (the buddleia family, the flowers of which are so attractive to butterflies). The fruit of the tree is about the size of a large apple but globular in shape. Under the hard rind, is a soft white pulp containing five, disc-shaped, seeds. The mother tincture is prepared from the dried seeds.

Nux vomica is often called 'the hangover remedy' because it can help to alleviate most of the symptoms of over indulgence. The seeds contain two alkaloids, Strychnine and Brucine, which are both poisonous. The taste, however, is very bitter so poisoning, fortunately, is rare.

Keynotes: Digestive upsets. Backache.

Uses: This remedy has a marked effect on the whole digestive system. It is, therefore, useful for ulcers in the mouth with a sour taste, accompanied by eructations (belches) from the stomach, which may be followed by nausea and vomiting.

Chronic and spasmodic bouts of colic, with much flatulence (wind) and discomfort, will benefit from doses of *Nux vomica*. Constipation, followed by diarrhoea after over-eating, and liver conditions, such as hepatitis, also indicate the use of *Nux vomica*. In animals, therefore, it is beneficial after scavenging causing colic and, also, in many cases of colitis.

The action of strychnine on the muscles, causing extreme spasms, means that it is also a useful remedy to consider when there is back pain and 'slipped disc.'

Modalities: Worse from dry, cold, and windy weather, after eating, and from lack of sleep or over-exertion. Better from warm and wet weather, while resting, in the evening, and after sleeping.

Suggested Potency: 6c or 30c.

Dosage: Every 2 hours up to 6 doses, then 4 times daily (every 4 hours) for as long as required, usually 2 to 4 days. In cases of colitis, it may be beneficial to take the remedy on a daily basis.

Additional Remedies: *Arsen. alb.* (see page 34) for acute vomiting and diarrhoea, *Colocynthis* (see page 55) for colic, *Merc. sol.* (see page 70) and *Podophyllum* (see page 76) for diarrhoea.

Anecdote: Tor was a large, and very impressive-looking, male Rottweiler who much enjoyed a good scavenge around the farmyard, frequently over-eating animal feed, that was lying about, and also horse and sheep droppings. Such over-indulgence caused bouts of obvious stomach-ache, abdominal discomfort with colicky symptoms, much flatus (passing wind) and then diarrhoea would inevitably follow. All these symptoms were well controlled with regular doses of *Nux vomica*.

Incidentally, his owner was also prone to over-indulgence with food and drink, causing similar symptoms with extreme irritability, so the same remedy suited both man and dog! (FH)

NUX VOMICA

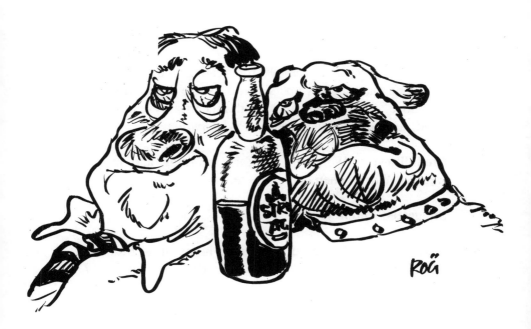

PODOPHYLLUM (Podophyllum peltatum)

Podophyllum belongs to the order Berberidaceae, although some botanists consider it to be a member of the order Ranunculaceae (the buttercup family), and it has close associations with both. It grows in the United States where it is known as the may apple or sometimes, because of its yellow egg-shaped fruits, as the wild lemon.

The remedy is prepared by making a tincture of the whole fresh plant including the roots and the fruit, both of which contain a resinous extract Podophyllin.

Keynotes: Enteritis (diarrhoea - gushing and offensive). Flatulence.

Uses: A very useful remedy for treating diarrhoea, even diarrhoea that may have persisted for some days. Morning diarrhoea, often accompanied with much flatus (passing of wind), usually responds well to *Podophyllum*.

Modalities: Worse in the early morning and in hot weather. Worse when babies are teething.

Suggested Potency: 6c.

Dosage: Initially, one dose every 2 hours up to 6 doses, then 4 times daily (approximately four hourly) for 5 to 7 days, as necessary.

Additional Remedies: *Argent. nit.* (see page 27) for diarrhoea, associated with anxiety. *Arsen. alb.* (see page 34) for acute vomiting and diarrhoea. *Merc. sol.* (see page 70) for diarrhoea with much pain and tenesmus (straining). Two other remedies, *Merc. corr.* (see page 100) and *Croton tig.*, (see page 99) are also worth considering when diarrhoea is a problem.

Anecdote: It was while visiting a house to attend a sick Bulldog that I first met the Mynah bird, Boris. Suddenly the room was filled with the awesome sound of a man's hacking cough! I turned round to find no man in the room, only Boris giving a wonderful imitation of the man of the house's hacking smoker's cough, with which he apparently started his day. At the same time, watery stools were gushing from his tail end.

The owner, Mrs Radley, had tried numerous different conventional medicines, including various antibiotics and anti-diarrhoea treatments, all without lasting success. At the time of my visit, Mrs Radley had no knowledge of homoeopathy but said she would be very happy to try a new approach to this persistent problem.

Boris started his treatment with *Podophyllum* the next day and, after quite a short time, he improved very nicely. He continued to 'cough' with great enthusiasm but his droppings, thankfully, returned to being normal and controllable. (FH)

PODOPHYLLUM

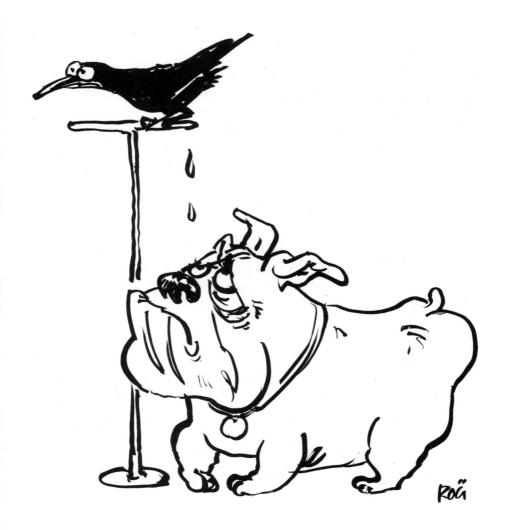

PULSATILLA (Pulsatilla nigricans)

This little plant belongs to the order Ranunculaceae (the buttercup family). It has several common names including meadow anemone, pasque flower and wind-flower. The name wind-flower well describes the plant itself and some of its actions. *Pulsatilla* is such an important remedy in homoeopathic medicine that it would be a mistake to omit it even from a simple book such as this.

The plant grows wild over much of the British countryside and Europe, especially on chalky soil, and it is also popular as a garden plant. It flowers in April and May and often, again, in September. The flowers are pretty, with purple petals and golden centres, but this delicate appearance should not deceive. The smell from the broken flowers or damaged leaves can bring on headaches, running eyes, and even fainting fits, and the juice on the skin may produce eczema or a burning sensation.

Keynotes: Catarrh. Reproductive problems. Toothache. Incontinence.

Uses: *Pulsatilla* is frequently used as a constitutional remedy (see page 16) where it can be useful for treating many ills. The name wind-flower reflects the action of this attractive plant blowing gently in the breeze. This, and the fact that it grows in clumps, imitates the variable and gregarious nature of the many patients who will benefit from this remedy. Toothache, accompanied by a dry mouth, sore gums, and an unpleasant taste in the mouth, may respond well from dosing with *Pulsatilla*. Chronic catarrh, earache with a creamy, often offensive-smelling discharge and sore eyes, frequently improve with *Pulsatilla*. *Pulsatilla*, when prescribed by a physician or veterinary surgeon, can be most useful in treating troubles associated with the birth process.

Modalities: Worse from heat, a stuffy room, lying on the left side and when resting. Better in the open air, especially cold dry air, and from gentle movement.

Suggested Potency: 30c.

Dosage: For acute cases, *Pulsatilla* may be given 3-4 times daily, for 5 to 7 days, until improvement is apparent. For toothache, use at the first aid rate (see page 14).

Additional Remedies: *Euphrasia* (see page 58) for eye problems and *Chamomilla* (see page 49) for toothache. The remedy, *Kali bich.* (see page 100) is also useful in many cases of catarrh and sinusitis.

Anecdotes:
1) Gerry, the smooth-haired miniature Dachshund, was 14 years old when he first had homoeopathic medicine. He had a number of chronic ailments, including persistent sinusitis with a running nose and eyes, bowel problems, skin troubles, to say nothing of various aches and pains

including a bad back. This prevented Gerry from climbing on his favourite chair or jumping on his owner's bed where he always slept, if possible, because Dachshunds do love to keep warm!

Pulsatilla turned out to be Gerry's constitutional remedy (see page 16) and he lived a happy life in good health until he was 20 years old. A long life indeed for any dog to live and, in this case, undoubtedly due in large measure to his gratifying response to homoeopathy. (FH)

2)   Miss Forbes had a small herd of 16 delightful pedigree Jersey cows. The cows were tied up for milking in a large, airy milking parlour, eight on each side. They still retained their horns because Miss Forbes did not hold with the practice of removing cows' horns.

Every day, each cow received its ration of dairy nuts, in a round washing-up bowl, and these were of various colours. When they had finished eating, and as a sign that they would like some more, they all picked up their bowls in their mouths and placed them upside down on their horns!

I was called, one day, to see Clementine, who was Miss Forbes' favourite cow, because she followed her everywhere. Clementine was off her food, not giving much milk, and she seemed to be rather sad, probably because she had, recently, been parted from her calf. There were no other signs of ill health and she was so obviously a constitutional *Pulsatilla* that I treated her with a few doses of this remedy and, in just a few days, Clementine was her cheery self again, much to the relief of Miss Forbes. (FH)

PULSATILLA

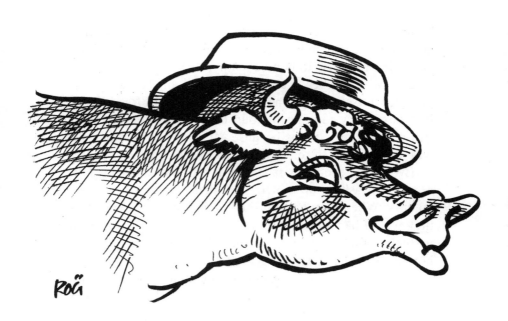

RHUS TOX. (Rhus toxicodendron)

Rhus tox. is often referred to as American poison ivy because it grows abundantly on the east coast of North America and in Canada. It is not found in the British Isles. *Rhus tox.* is a member of the family Anarcardiaceae.

This is one of the major medicines used in homoeopathy and, after *Arnica*, is probably the next most well known to the general public. The plant trails along the ground and then grows up around anything it can find as a support, in the same manner as our native ivy. The remedy is prepared from freshly gathered leaves just before the plant is due to flower. The active principle, thought to be a phenol, is so irritant that touching or even just brushing against the leaves can set off acute and intense irritation.

Keynotes: Arthritis. Rheumatism. Skin irritation. (Always better for movement).

Uses: There are two principal uses for this remedy:

1) Joint and muscular pain: Such pains may be caused by sprains or strains or more severe conditions, such as arthritis and/or rheumatism. Many such conditions will respond to *Rhus tox.* but it is important to remember that this remedy works well in conditions where there is some improvement, be it only slight, with movement.

2) Skin problems: Acute skin irritation, particularly with blister formation and an intense desire to rub or scratch the affected area. This is an important treatment for

shingles and seems to work most effectively if given when the symptoms first appear.

Modalities: Worse from cold, cold winds, and the combination of wet and cold. Worse at night and during rest, whether standing, sitting or lying. There is, initially, pain on first movement which then eases slightly as movement continues. Better, in dry warm weather, and from moving about. Better from wrapping up warmly, warm applications applied locally, and from massage of the affected parts. (Compare *Bryonia* (see page 40) - worse for any movement; better for application of cold.)

Suggested Potency: 6c or 30c. *Rhus tox.* for joint pain, etc seems to work better in a 6c given frequently (up to 4 times daily), for the elderly, and in a 30c for the younger patient. Skin problems, especially shingles, respond well to the 30c.

Dosage: One dose 4-6 times daily, as necessary, reducing to 1-4 doses daily when improvement is apparent.

Additional Remedies: *Bryonia* (see page 40) where any pain or discomfort is made worse by moving about. *Ruta* (see page 101) if muscle tissues are involved. *Hypericum* (see page 67) for muscular back pain.

Anecdote: Drummond, the Labrador, was a marvellous gun dog, instantly obedient to every command from his master and, with a lovely soft mouth, he was the ideal retriever. Unfortunately Drummond, at nine years old, was getting stiff and lethargic and it looked as if his working days were over.

Drummond did not respond to conventional treatments which upset him and caused vomiting and diarrhoea. Homoeopathic assistance was sought and regular treatment with "Rusty Tox", as his owner called it, gave Drummond two more shooting seasons (and how he loved his work!), followed by a long and pain-free retirement. (FH)

RHUS TOX.

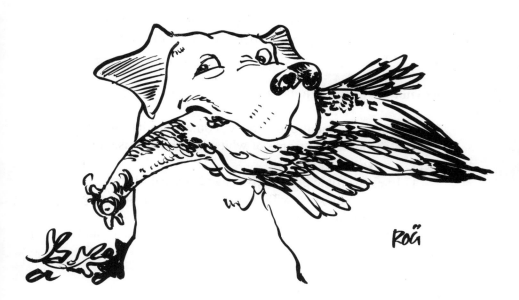

SILICEA (Silica)

The everyday names for *Silicea* are sand (sandstone), flint, and quartz ('quartz' watches and clocks are activated by quartz crystals). *Silicea* occurs in nature as the chemical substance, silicon dioxide, and is found everywhere, on land and under the sea.

This apparently inert mineral has little application in conventional medicine but, once again, like other unusual substances included in this book, such as *Argent. nit., Hepar sulph.,* and *Merc. sol., Silicea* has an important action in homoeopathy. Strangely too, when used as a constitutional remedy (see page 16), the characteristics of a *'Silicea'* patient reflect the properties of sand, being normally of a quiet and rather lethargic, inactive, nature. However, once roused (as in a sandstorm for instance), the *'Silicea'* personality may become violent and even destructive.

Keynotes: Chronic, long-lasting, conditions.

Uses: *Silicea,* as mentioned above, comes into its own for treating chronic cases, some of which may have existed for weeks or even months.

1) Eyes: Chronic conjunctivitis and corneal ulcer.

2) Nose: Sinusitis with frequent bouts of sneezing, irritation of the nose and sore nasal bones.

3) Bowels: Chronic, alternating diarrhoea and constipation.

4) Bones and Joints: Pains, with much stiffness and discomfort, when first moving from rest. Chronic cramp spasms.

5) Skin: Long lasting skin conditions, often accompanied by sepsis and pus formation (as with pimples and boils), and delayed healing. Splitting, brittle, malformed nails should also respond to treatment with *Silicea*.

6) In addition, *Silicea* can help to eliminate from the body things such as thorns, splinters of wood, metal or glass, which may have been lodged somewhere for a while.

Modalities: Worse at the time of the new moon. Worse in the morning, from cold air and weather, from thunderstorms and lying on the painful side. Better from warmth, wrapping up well, and in the summer.

Suggested Potency: 30c works well for most conditions but 6c, given over a long period, may be called for when treating chronic skin ulcers and ulcers on the cornea (or front) of the eye.

Dosage: 3 times a day for 7 to 10 days. For longer term chronic treatment, the 6c potency, taken twice daily, would be appropriate.

Additional Remedies: *Hepar sulph.* (see page 64) for infections. *Bryonia* (see page 40) and *Rhus tox.* (see page 83) for arthritis and rheumatism. *Euphrasia* (see page 58) and *Symphytum* (see page 93) and *Ledum* (see page 100) for the eyes. *Arsen. alb.* (see page 34) and *Sulphur* (see page 90) for the skin.

Anecdote: Rupert was a fine-looking, big, crossbred Hunter, impressive to behold in every way except for his poor feet! The horn of the hooves was very dry and brittle and pieces kept breaking away, giving a very ragged appearance. It came to the point where the blacksmith was in despair and declared that he was not sure if it would be possible to put shoes on Rupert at all the next time, that he was due to be shod, which would be in a couple of months time. The horn was in such a poor state, it was well nigh impossible to get the nails to hold the shoes in place without fragments coming away.

Rupert was referred for homoeopathy because his chronic sinusitis and running nose would not respond to conventional therapy and *Silicea* was prescribed for this condition. It was a pleasing bonus, and a surprise too, when his feet improved as well as his sinusitis. (FH)

SILICEA

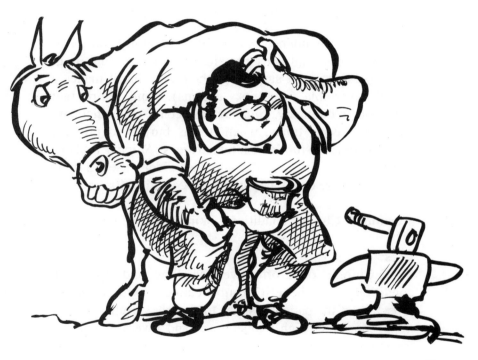

roü

SULPHUR (Sulphur)

Sulphur or 'flowers of sulphur', as it is often called, can be made in the laboratory by sublimation, but it is the naturally occurring element that is used in homoeopathy. *Sulphur* is yellow and rock-like but, after it has been burned, it forms a yellow, crystal-like powder; hence the 'flowers'.

Sulphur is contained in our bodies naturally and forms part of the essential body proteins and so is present in all our tissues. It is not surprising, therefore, that it makes a useful, variable (in its actions), and important homoeopathic remedy. *Sulphur* has been used medicinally since very early times, when it was burned to produce noxious fumes to fumigate infected areas. *Sulphur* is also a constituent of Epsom salts and the widely used Sulpha drugs that were developed in the 1930s and 1940s.

Keynotes: Chronic conditions. Skin problems. Fevers.

Uses:

1) Chronic, often offensively-smelling, and septic skin conditions will benefit from treatment with *Sulphur*, especially if the patient dislikes too much warmth.

2) Persistent high temperatures and fevers, which are frequently caused by virus infections, can be controlled by *Sulphur* treatment. Conventional medicine to date has little to offer, to treat virus infections, and it is gratifying to see the persistent high temperature coming down, after dosing with *Sulphur*.

Modalities: Worse from heat of any sort, when standing, from the warmth of the bed, and from washing or bathing. 11am in the morning seems to be a particularly bad time. Better in dry, not too warm weather, and from lying on the right side.

Suggested Potency: 6c for skin problems over a period of time and 30c, or higher, to reduce temperatures. It is worth noting that often the best results with *Sulphur*, particularly using the potencies higher than 30c, are obtained under the guidance of a trained health professional.

Dosage: 2-4 times daily for variable periods of time, according to the condition being treated, is recommended. Seek advice, if in doubt.

Additional Remedies: For skin problems that persist, it is advisable to seek professional advice. For fevers, *Aconite* (see page 21) and *Belladonna* (see page 37) may be indicated.

Anecdote: I often recall a talk on constitutional remedies (see page 16) given by the Bristol homoeopathic physician, Dr Hughes-Games, in which he demonstrated, with photographs, some of the different 'homoeopathic types'.

One picture showed the front garden of a house devoid of lawn and flowers but completely filled with broken-down cars, old motor bikes, washing-machines, and other assorted bits of junk. Such untidy and slovenly habits often denote the *'Sulphur'* type.

Recently, I called at just such a dwelling to see a sick dog. The smell of 'dog', and goodness knows what else, that greeted me as the door was opened was quite overpowering.

Thumper, as "the trying to be a Labrador" was called, was very overweight, dirty, unkempt and covered in nasty sores all over his body. I have to say that the owners did not look in much better shape. Thumper was lying on the cold tiles in the kitchen and apparently shunned the heat whenever he could (see Modalities above). I treated him over a period of time with *Sulphur* and he responded well. I cannot speak, however, for his owners or the garden! (FH)

SULPHUR

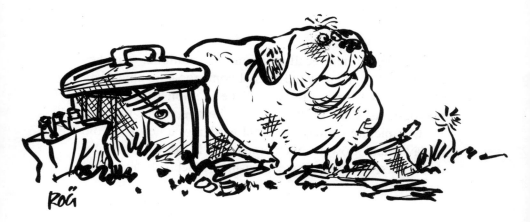

ROü

SYMPHYTUM (Symphytum officinale)

Symphytum belongs to the family Boraginaceae, which also contains the 'forget-me-not' group of plants. The common name is comfrey and folklore names are 'boneset' and 'knitbone'. This remedy should not be confused with herbal forms of 'knitbone', with which there have been problems because of side effects.

This remedy is included because it is useful but, also, fascinating with its history as a medical herb. As far back as mediaeval times, the root of the comfrey plant was ground into a thick paste and placed round fractured bones, where it soon hardened and formed a type of cast, rather as plaster of paris is used today.

Keynotes: Fractures. Eye injuries.

Uses: In homoeopathic potency, it can be taken by mouth and helps fractures, especially those that are slow to unite, to knit together, or where there has been surgical intervention eg. dental operations.

Injuries to the eye, from severe blows or knocks, respond well to treatment with *Symphytum* which is acknowledged to be one of the best remedies for traumatic injuries.

Modalities: This is the only remedy in the book with no significant modalities to help selection of a particular remedy. For more information about modalities, see page 17.

Suggested Potency: 30c.

Dosage: One dose, 3 times daily, for a period of 10 days. Clinical experience has shown that it can be beneficial to repeat the course of treatment after 2 weeks.

Additional Remedies: *Arnica* (see page 30) for general injuries. *Euphrasia* (see page 58) for certain conditions of the eye. *Ledum* (see page 100) for eye injuries.

Anecdote: Esmerelda was a goat and a very special pet in the Fraser household. She was born on the smallholding, and was a great favourite with the younger children and followed them everywhere.

Esmerelda was only six months old when she fell off a wall and broke her front leg below the knee. The Vet set it in a plaster cast and everybody who called at the house signed their name on it because Esmerelda was always about when visitors arrived. Unfortunately, because she was such an active little goat, the fracture just would not heal and allow the bones to knit together properly.

After some weeks, it looked as if the 'unmentionable' might be the only solution. A kind friend suggested that homoeopathy might be able to help, so Esmerelda arrived at the surgery as a referral. Two 10-day courses of *Symphytum*, with a space of a fortnight between them, did the trick.

As far as I know, some few years on, Esmerelda is still doing fine, providing milk for the household, having babies of her own, and is still very much one of the family. (FH)

SYMPHYTUM

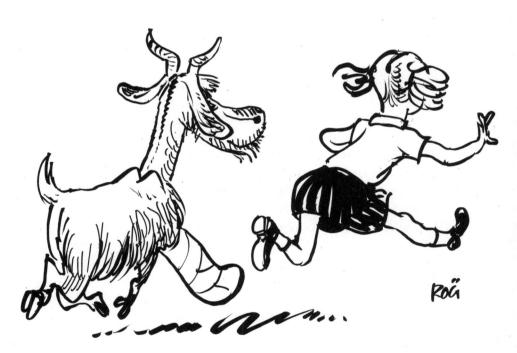

URTICA (Urtica Urens)

Urtica is the common stinging nettle and so this useful remedy is found growing literally everywhere. It belongs to its own family, the Urticaceae.

The remedy is prepared from the fresh plant of the small stinging nettle when it is in flower. The properties of the small nettle are similar, if not identical, to those of the common nettle, Urtica dioica, although the active ingredients may differ slightly.

Keynotes: Skin conditions. Burns and scalds. Nettle-rash (Urticaria).

Uses: The value of this remedy, in the treatment of acute burns and scalds, cannot be over-emphasised. The remedy may be given by mouth, and also the cream or ointment, which is prepared from a mixture of *Hypericum* (see page 67) and *Urtica*, should be applied liberally and immediately. Urticaria (nettle-rash, heat-rash, or hives) with intolerable itching, as after brushing against nettles, will also benefit from treatment with *Urtica*. In addition, *Urtica* can be used to treat oedema and gout.

Modalities: Worse from touch, water, cool moist air, and in the snow.

Suggested Potency: 6c, or 30c for very severe cases.

96

Dosage: For acute burns and scalds, repeated doses, at intervals of 15-20 minutes, may be given up to a total of 6, or until relief of symptoms is evident.

For other conditions, a dose given 3 times daily, for a few days, should be sufficient.

Additional Remedies: *Apis mel.*(see page 24) for stings. *Belladonna* (see page 37) and *Cantharis* (see page 43) are also effective for skin symptoms resulting from burns, including sunburn.

Anecdote: Janice, our nurse/receptionist suffered badly from 'prickly heat' (heat-rash) when the weather was really hot. Janice was particularly anxious because she was about to get married, and the honeymoon was to be in the height of summer in a south Mediterranean country.

When I heard of her concern, I supplied her with a number of homoeopathic remedies to take with her, including *Urtica*. The honeymoon went well, it appears, and not a sign of the dreaded 'prickly heat'.

Now, there are two sweet little children but I'm not certain if *Urtica* had anything to do with that! (FH)

URTICA

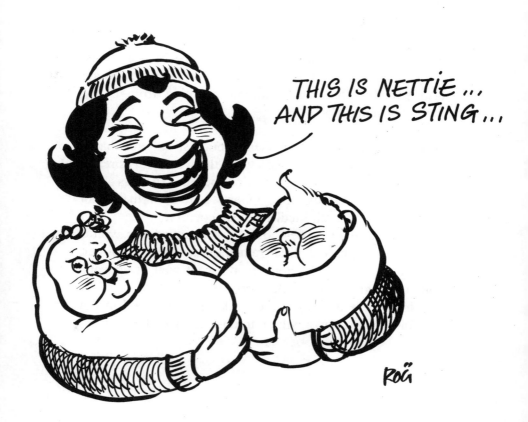

ADDITIONAL REMEDIES

Brief details are given here of the 12 additional remedies that are mentioned in the text, but do not have their own entry.

For suggested dosage of these remedies, see levels of treatment and dose regimes (pages 12-16).

BELLIS PERENNIS
The common daisy, in a potency of 6c, may be used for sprains with much soreness, wrist pain, and for giddiness in elderly people.

BORAX
A low potency of 3c, or even 3x, seems to work well when loud noises due to thunderstorms, fireworks or gunshots are the problem. The remedy may be repeated several times, at intervals of 15-20 minutes, if it seems to be beneficial.

COFFEA CRUDA
Coffea is, in fact, made from unroasted coffee. It is helpful in a potency of 30c for extreme excitability, intolerance to pain and for unusual activity of the body and brain. *Coffea* is also included in homoeopathic remedies for insomnia (sleeplessness).

CROTON TIG.
Croton tig., in a 30c potency, is a useful alternative to *Podophyllum* (see page 76), when there is copious watery

diarrhoea with much straining and gurgling intestinal noises. The condition may be worsened by drinking or even while eating.

KALI BICH.

Kali bich., in a 30c potency, may be useful when there are yellow discharges from the eyes and nostrils and also, possibly, from the ears. It is often indicated and effective in cases of chronic catarrh and sinusitis.

LACHESIS

The venom of the deadly Bushmaster snake is used, sometimes, for treating jealousy in both humans and animals and is best left for the Professional to prescribe.

LEDUM PAL.

Marsh tea, as it is known, is a small shrub resembling the tea plant and, in a similar way, can be used as a drink. It is an important remedy for treating puncture wounds and animal bites. It follows *Arnica* (see page 30) well, when blood patches persist under the skin. Use in the 30c potency.

MERC. CORR.

A valuable remedy when the symptoms described under *Merc. sol.* (see page 70) are very severe. This is particularly the case when there is dysentery with blood in the stool and excessive straining, with cutting pains, and an offensive odour. Use the 30c potency.

PETROLEUM

This remedy is prepared from crude petroleum and, like *Tabacum* (see below), is a useful 'travel remedy' to try, if treatment with *Cocculus* (see page 52) does not prove successful. Use the 30c potency.

RUTA

This is prepared from rue, a common hedgerow plant, that has been used medicinally as a herb since ancient times. *Ruta* is a useful alternative to *Rhus tox.* (see page 83) when there is overstrain of muscles and tendons. The pains seem worse when resting and lying down, and also when walking out of doors. This is where it differs from *Rhus tox.* Use the 6c potency.

STAPHYSAGRIA

A remedy useful for resentment but, like *Lachesis* (see above), is best left for the Professional to prescribe.

TABACUM

The 'tobacco plant' is another useful 'travel remedy'. *Tabacum* can also be helpful to overcome giddiness and nausea with icy coldness, deathly pallor and cold sweat. This makes it a particularly useful remedy for seasickness. Use in the 30c potency.

TOPICAL PREPARATIONS

These preparations are usually applied, sparingly, to the skin once or twice daily, until the symptoms subside, and can be used in conjunction with other homoeopathic, or orthodox, treatments. They are extremely effective. There is little difference between the products from various manufacturers although, just occasionally, the base being used can cause a slight allergic reaction.

a) Ointments and creams.

Ointments and creams are not sterile and should not be applied where the skin is broken. Under these circumstances, oral medication should be used.

Examples of preparations containing single ingredients:

Arnica: Applied after bruising. Can also be used for aching muscles after prolonged activity or an accident.

Calendula: Excellent in the treatment of minor skin abrasions.

Hamamelis: Often combined with other remedies in the treatment of haemorrhoids, *Hamamelis* is also used alone in the topical treatment of varicose conditions on the legs.

Hypericum: May be combined with *Calendula*, with which it shares many applications. It is indicated for painful crush injuries, especially when fingers, toes or paws are involved, but not when the skin is extensively broken.

Rhus tox: Useful where there is deep arthritic-type joint pain, either alone or as an adjunct to treatment by mouth.

Ruta: Applied in cases of soft tissue injuries, torn tendons, split ligaments and, possibly, synovitis. It is sometimes used in conjunction with *Rhus tox*.

Thuja: An effective treatment for warts and verrucae. A good starting point but, if treatment is ineffective, can be combined with oral therapy or mother tincture.

Urtica: It can be used in cases of urticarial-type eruptions, as well as to treat 'prickly heat' rashes.

Examples of mixed ointments/creams:

Burn ointment: Contains several ingredients, but mainly *Cantharis*. Confers rapid relief after scalds and burns. Also useful for sunburn.

Haemorrhoid ointment: A mixture of *Aesculus*, *Hamamelis* and *Paeonia* mother tinctures. One manufacturer supplies tubes with handy applicators.

Hypericum and Calendula is widely known as Hypercal® (A. Nelson & Co). This is one of the most frequently used preparations, combining the indications of its two constituents.

Other preparations.

This category includes Tea tree cream, Vitamin E cream and Bach Rescue Cream®. Weleda have a range of branded topical preparations.

b) Lotions, liniments and oils.

Arnica, Calendula and *Hypericum* are three remedies used most frequently in these forms. *Rhus tox.* and *Ruta* may be used as a liniment or oil. *Verbascum* oil (also known as 'Mullein') is used as ear drops to soften wax and treat otalgia.

c) Mother tinctures.

Once again, it is recommended that mother tinctures are applied, topically, only when the skin is unbroken. They may be diluted with tepid water.

Arnica (bruises), **Calendula and Hypericum** (superficial abrasions) can be used in the bath. Gargles, mouthwashes and lotions can be made by placing 5 drops of mother tincture in a cup of warm water. They can be applied to the skin, providing there is no deep wound.

Ledum is suitable for insect bites - particularly puncture wounds.

Paeonia is effective in treating externally protruding haemorrhoids.

Phytolacca might be used in mastitis, although the remedy is more effective when given orally in potentised tablet form.

THE BACH FLOWER REMEDIES

A range of remedies derived from flowers was discovered by the English bacteriologist and physician Edward Bach, who was born in Birmingham in 1886. Dr Bach (whose name is usually pronounced 'Batch', although the gutteral 'ch', as in the Scottish 'loch', is also used) became a homoeopath, but found the complexity of homoeopathic prescribing rather difficult to master. He took his holidays in Wales and Norfolk, enjoying long walks in the countryside. It is claimed that he was intuitively drawn towards certain wild flowers that he was able to associate with particular emotions.

The Bach Flower remedies comprise a total of 38 medicines considered by Dr Bach to be sufficient to treat each of the most common negative moods that afflict mankind.

Although Bach flower remedies have come to be included under the homoeopathic umbrella, they are not really homoeopathic for a number of reasons, of which the following are examples:

- They have not undergone provings.
- Prescribing is based on an accurate perception of the mental state, rather than matching symptoms to a drug picture, as in classical homoeopathy.
- They have a wide spectrum of activity and are not known to be negatively affected by such agents as tea or coffee.

Flower remedies are becoming increasingly popular, and are stocked by many pharmacies and health food shops.

One of the difficulties experienced, when using these remedies, is that mental symptoms can change during treatment. As a patient feels better, there is a strong likelihood that a different flower remedy will be more appropriate. In order to deal with this problem, there is an extremely useful combination of five Bach Flower remedies, known as 'Rescue Remedy'®. It was so named for its stabilising and calming effect on the emotions, during a crisis, and it has considerable applications in veterinary medicine, especially where animals are suffering from the effects of stress.

The remedy comprises:

Cherry plum (for fear of not being able to cope, in humans),

Clematis (for unconsciousness or the 'detached' sensations that often accompany trauma),

Impatiens (for impatience, agitation),

Rock rose (for terror), and

Star of Bethlehem (for the after-effects of shock).

This remedy can be used in place of *Arnica* (see page 30), when the mental symptoms resulting from an accident, or overwork, are more evident than the physical.

Owners are instructed to add two drops of the Bach Flower remedy to their pet's drinking bowl. If the animal is not drinking, then two drops of the remedy may be placed in the mouth. 'Rescue Remedy' is also available as a cream that can be applied to skin conditions resulting from anxiety.

THE END - OR THE BEGINNING?

Homoeopathy is no different from conventional medicine (sometimes called 'allopathy') in that it does not ALWAYS provide relief or a cure. Some conditions simply do not respond.

One thing is certain, however. Homoeopathic remedies are perfectly safe in infancy, during pregnancy, and in later life. Further, they will not interfere with any existing or subsequent medication. The only harm you can do is to try and treat a condition beyond your capability. This may result in extending the time that discomfort has to be suffered by the patient or, even worse, it may mean you miss a much more serious condition.

So, one final word of caution. Remember, this book is designed to help you treat **simple self-limiting conditions**. **YOU SHOULD NOT REDUCE OR DISCONTINUE ANY PRESCRIBED ORTHODOX MEDICATION OR ATTEMPT TO TREAT COMPLICATED LONG-STANDING CONDITIONS WITHOUT FIRST SEEKING ADVICE FROM YOUR DOCTOR OR VETERINARIAN.**

The only way to convince yourself that homoeopathy works is to use it. This may be the end of the book, but we hope that it is also the start of your introduction to a fascinating new world of healing!

We know that animals cannot read, but people can, so please spread the word about homoeopathy, the gentle art of healing, to your friends and, of course, to your pets as well.

CONCLUSION

Francis: Do you feel that we have achieved our aim, Steven?

Steven: At the risk of being big-headed, I will say yes, I think we have. We've shown that homoeopathic remedies can be used in everyday situations and, with the help of some stories from our case books and some pictures which will jog the memory, we hope that this will enable people to use remedies to treat simple self-limiting type conditions.

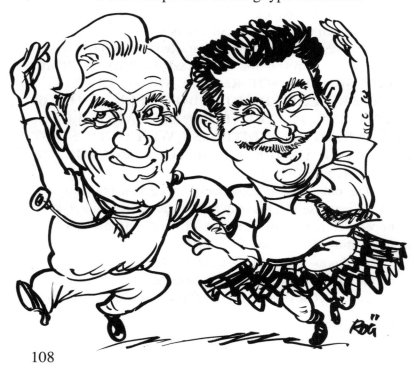

SELECT BIBLIOGRAPHY

Boericke, W.   Materia Medica with Repertory.
              Boericke & Runyon 1927.
Clarke, J.H.   The Prescriber.
              Health Science Press (9th Ed) 1972.
Gibson, D.   Studies of Homoeopathic Remedies.
              Beaconsfield Press 1987.
Gibson, D.   First Aid Homoeopathy in accidents and
              ailments.
              British Homoeopathic Association 1993.
Hunter, F.E.   Homoeopathic First Aid Treatment for Pets.
              Thorsons Publishers Ltd 1988.
              (First publ. as "Before the Vet Calls" 1984)
Kayne, S.   Homoeopathic Pharmacy.
              Churchill Livingstone 1997.
Macleod, G.   Veterinary Materia Medica & Clinical
              Repertory.
              C.W. Daniel Co Ltd 1983.
Tyler, M.L.   Homoeopathic Drug Pictures.
              Health Science Press 1970.
Wolff, H.G.   Homoeopathic Medicine for Dogs.
              Thorsons Publishers Ltd 1984.

THE BRITISH HOMOEOPATHIC ASSOCIATION

Founded in 1902, the BHA is a registered charity managed by an independent council.

We are honoured to have Queen Elizabeth, The Queen Mother, as our Royal Patron.

If you are interested in homoeopathy, then supporting the BHA is the natural choice for you. For a modest annual sum, you can help the development of homoeopathy as well as benefit from a wide range of member services including a copy of our journal 'Homoeopathy', which is sent to your home six times a year, and use of our extensive library.

The BHA keeps up-to-date address lists of homoeopathic doctors and veterinary surgeons, as well as lists of homoeopathic clinics and hospitals.

On receipt of a stamped, self-addressed envelope, an information pack, including a membership form, and any list required will be sent to you, by return of post.

The BHA also stocks a wide range of books on homoeopathy, as well as the homoeopathic treatment of animals, all of which can be purchased at the BHA office or ordered by post, enclosing a cheque made out to British Homoeopathic Association Enterprises Ltd. The current book-list is included in the aforementioned information pack.

INDEX

114